Dental Caries Perspectives - A Collection of Thoughtful Essays

Edited by Ana Cláudia Rodrigues Chibinski

Published in London, United Kingdom

Dental Caries Perspectives - A Collection of Thoughtful Essays
http://dx.doi.org/10.5772/intechopen.110999
Edited by Ana Cláudia Rodrigues Chibinski

Contributors
Ana Cláudia Rodrigues Chibinski, Anfal Mohammad Muhammad Alqussier, Anna Bárbara Maluf, Krishnaa Sudeep, Larissa Yumi Ito, Letícia Maira Wambier, Mayara Vitorino Gevert, Sudeep Sarathchandran, Sukumaran Anil, Thomas Davidson, Urvashi Bhimjibhai Sodvadia, Vishnupriya K. Sweety, Vitória Monteiro

First published in London, United Kingdom, 2024 by IntechOpen
IntechOpen is the global imprint of INTECHOPEN LIMITED, registered in England and Wales, registration number: 11086078, 167-169 Great Portland Street, London, W1W 5PF, United Kingdom

British Library Cataloguing-in-Publication Data
A catalogue record for this book is available from the British Library

Additional hard and PDF copies can be obtained from orders@intechopen.com

Dental Caries Perspectives - A Collection of Thoughtful Essays
Edited by Ana Cláudia Rodrigues Chibinski
p. cm.

This title is part of the Dentistry Book Series, Volume 16
Topic: Oral Health
Series Editor: Sergio Alexandre Gehrke
Topic Editor: Sandra Marinho and Esra Guzeldemir-Akcakanat

Print ISBN 978-0-85014-111-5
Online ISBN 978-0-85014-112-2
eBook (PDF) ISBN 978-0-85014-113-9
ISSN 2631-6218

For EU product safety concerns:
IN TECH d.o.o., Prolaz Marije Krucifikse Kozulić 3, 51000 Rijeka, Croatia,
info@intechopen.com or visit our website at intechopen.com.

IntechOpen Book Series

Dentistry

Volume 16

Aims and Scope of the Series

This book series will offer a comprehensive overview of recent research trends as well as clinical applications within different specialties of dentistry. Topics will include overviews of the health of the oral cavity, from prevention and care to different treatments for the rehabilitation of problems that may affect the organs and/or tissues present. The different areas of dentistry will be explored, with the aim of disseminating knowledge and providing readers with new tools for the comprehensive treatment of their patients with greater safety and with current techniques. Ongoing issues, recent advances, and future diagnostic approaches and therapeutic strategies will also be discussed. This series of books will focus on various aspects of the properties and results obtained by the various treatments available, whether preventive or curative.

Meet the Series Editor

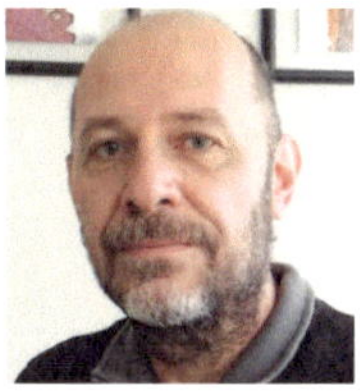

Dr. Sergio Alexandre Gehrke is a doctorate holder in two fields. The first is a Ph.D. in Cellular and Molecular Biology from the Pontificia Catholic University, Porto Alegre, Brazil, in 2010 and the other is an International Ph.D. in Bioengineering from the Universidad Miguel Hernandez, Elche/Alicante, Spain, obtained in 2020. In 2018, he completed a postdoctoral fellowship in Materials Engineering in the NUCLEMAT of the Pontificia Catholic University, Porto Alegre, Brazil. He is currently the Director of the Postgraduate Program in Implantology of the Bioface/UCAM/PgO (Montevideo, Uruguay), Director of the Cathedra of Biotechnology of the Catholic University of Murcia (Murcia, Spain), an Extraordinary Full Professor of the Catholic University of Murcia (Murcia, Spain) as well as the Director of the private center of research Biotecnos – Technology and Science (Montevideo, Uruguay). Applied biomaterials, cellular and molecular biology, and dental implants are among his research interests. He has published several original papers in renowned journals. In addition, he is also a Collaborating Professor in several Postgraduate programs at different universities all over the world.

Meet the Volume Editor

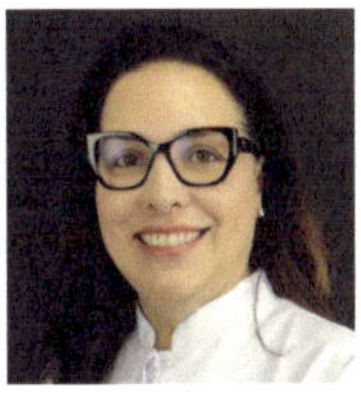

Professor Ana Cláudia Rodrigues Chibinski is an associate professor in the Department of Dentistry, State University of Ponta Grossa, Brazil. She obtained her specialist title in pediatric dentistry from the Federal University of Paraná, Brazil, and holds the title of specialist in health education from the Federal University of Rio Grande do Sul, Brazil. She earned both a master's degree and a Ph.D. in Dental Clinics from the State University of Ponta Grossa. Her Ph.D. was conferred after defending a doctoral thesis titled "In vivo evaluation of changes in infected dentin from deciduous teeth after minimally invasive restorative treatment." With extensive experience in clinical pediatric dentistry across both private and public sectors, her primary research interests lie in minimally invasive dentistry, restorative materials, and systematic reviews in *Pediatric Dentistry*. She is a member of the Brazilian Dental Association and the Brazilian Association of Pediatric Dentistry. She has published more than eighty peer-reviewed papers. Additionally, Dr. Chibinski is a frequent lecturer at national and international events.

Contents

Preface

Despite advancements in oral health care, dental caries continue to be a significant public health issue worldwide. As clinicians and researchers, we are acutely aware of the impact that caries can have on individuals' oral health and overall well-being. Therefore, it is with great pleasure and humility that we present this publication.

However, it is important to emphasize that the intention behind this book was not to provide exhaustive coverage of every aspect of dental caries study. Instead, it serves as a platform for authors to share their unique perspectives, experiences, and findings, contributing to a broader understanding of the multifaceted nature of caries research. Also, as we navigate the ever-evolving landscape of dental science, it is essential to acknowledge that this book represents a snapshot in time—a culmination of our collective knowledge and understanding up to this point. Dentistry is a dynamic field, constantly evolving with new research findings and technological advancements. Therefore, this book should be viewed as a catalyst for ongoing learning and exploration. In the diagnosis of caries, for instance, we aim to underscore the importance of meticulous diagnosis, highlighting the new methods and technologies available to clinicians. We also emphasize the importance of adopting minimally invasive dentistry approaches, such as selective caries removal and remineralization of incipient lesions, to improve the quality of the treatment and preserve dental tissue. We believe that effective preventive and therapeutic strategies are built through a better understanding of the dynamics of caries, which results in optimal patient care and long-term oral health outcomes.

Each chapter represents a distinct viewpoint, focusing on specific aspects. As such, readers should approach this book as a collection of diverse viewpoints rather than a comprehensive guide to dental caries. We acknowledge that there are many areas left unexplored. Nonetheless, we believe that the varied insights presented within these pages will enrich readers' understanding of dental caries and inspire further exploration and discussion within the field.

This book is the culmination of collaborative efforts from esteemed professors and researchers from around the world. Their dedication to advancing the field of dentistry and their willingness to share their expertise have been instrumental in bringing this project to fruition. We are immensely grateful for their contributions and recognize the invaluable role they have played in shaping this book.

Finally, we hope that this book will serve as a valuable resource for clinicians, researchers, and students alike, inspiring critical thinking and encouraging the seeking out of new knowledge and innovative solutions.

Ana Cláudia Rodrigues Chibinski
Departament of Dentistry,
State University of Ponta Grossa,
Ponta Grossa, Paraná, Brazil

Section 1

Introduction

Chapter 1

Introductory Chapter: Contemporary Concepts in Cariology

Ana Cláudia Rodrigues Chibinski

1. Introduction

Untreated tooth decay remains one of the most prevalent diseases around the world. Data from 1990 to 2019 showed that there were 3.09 billion of new cases of untreated dental caries in permanent teeth (48.00% increase) and 1.15 billion in deciduous teeth (11.74% increase) [1]. This accounts for approximately 44% of the world's population.

Tooth decay is defined as a non-infectious, biofilm/sugar-dependent disease with multifactorial etiology and clinically manifests as lesions resulting from a process of mineral loss in the dental structure. Through a process of dysbiosis or imbalance, the microorganisms present in the oral environment become pathological, thus being responsible for the development of tooth decay. For many years, it was believed that *Streptococcus mutans* were largely responsible for this, but studies proved that this group represents only a small fraction of the bacterial community present in the biofilm responsible for disease process. Therefore, dental caries cannot be considered an infectious and contagious disease, since the ecological plaque hypothesis showed that tooth decay is not caused by a specific type of microorganism, but rather by the result of a change in the microbiota of the biofilm to more cariogenic species.

The oral microbiome has a symbiotic relationship with the host, and the presence of available sucrose in the mouth is a decisive factor to initiate the caries process. The American Academy of Pediatric Dentistry (AAPD) already cited that high frequency of sugar intake is one of the main risk factors for tooth decay, in addition to other variables such as low saliva flow, visible plaque on the tooth surface, use of dental appliances, health problems, sociodemographic factors, access to health care, among others.

Another factor that increases the risk of disease development and progression is the presence of alterations in dental structure, such as enamel defects, which hinder oral hygiene and biofilm control by the patient. Socio-economic-behavioral factors should also be considered as risk factors for tooth decay, as they can interfere with the course of the disease. Inadequate housing conditions, low income, low education, and habits that do not take into account the necessary oral health care also pose greater risks for the onset and development of the disease [2].

The risk factors and protective factors should be analyzed in each individual in a way that favors the assessment, prevention, and individualized intervention for each patient.

IntechOpen

2. How a carious lesion is formed?

In a very simplistic way, a carious lesion begins with a mineral loss in the hard dental tissues due to the imbalance in the demineralization and remineralization processes that physiologically occur in the mouth. Bacteria present in dental biofilm metabolize fermentable carbohydrates ingested by the individual and consequently produce organic acids (mainly lactic acid), leading to microbial adaptation that results in the selection of acidogenic microorganisms. With the predominance of these microorganisms, the oral pH decreases, and the oral environment becomes acidic. Therefore, an imbalance in the ion exchange between the tooth and saliva is settled [3].

For enamel, the lesion occurs when the pH reaches the critical level, which is below 5.5 in the absence of fluoride and 4.5 in the presence of fluoride. In this situation, there will be a breakdown of hydroxyapatite crystals, and the biofilm/enamel interface will become supersaturated with ions compared to saliva, leading to a loss of minerals to the environment, a process known as demineralization.

If the cariogenic biofilm is disorganized by toothbrushing, for instance, and there is no more available sucrose in the oral cavity, the acid production will cease and the pH will return to neutrality. The buffering action of saliva helps in this process. As a consequence, the biofilm/enamel interface, which was previously hypersaturated due to mineral loss, will now become undersaturated compared to saliva and will receive back calcium, phosphate, and hydroxyl ions, a process known as remineralization.

The process of demineralization and remineralization (DE-RE) mentioned above occurs daily in a subclinical manner in the oral cavity of all individuals. However, in cases of imbalance, such as lack of oral hygiene and high frequency of sugar consumption, this process remains much longer in the loss phase than in the mineral gain phase. If this movement is not interrupted, the acids will increase the porosity of the enamel, and there will be a widening between the spaces of hydroxyapatite crystals, resulting initially in a rough and opaque enamel surface, clinically seen as a white spot lesion. In cases where this process persists for a longer period, there will be a breakdown of the superficial layer of the lesion, resulting in a cavity.

3. Diagnosis

Timely and accurate diagnosis, as in all diseases, favors the definition of an effective treatment plan and improves the prognosis. Dental caries diagnosis involves the evaluation of signs and symptoms presented by the patient, but mainly the modifying factors involved in the onset and progression of tooth decay. Currently, the focus should no longer be solely on treating carious lesions or cavities, but rather on treating tooth decay as a whole disease.

The first step in diagnosis should be conducting an anamnesis to collect and assess the etiological or protective factors related to the disease. After completing the entire anamnesis, a clinical examination is necessary, during which all dental surfaces are evaluated for the detection and characterization of carious lesions.

It is important to note that there is no single method capable of assessing the onset of the disease. Therefore, we use various strategies to gather information and categorize the patient into a group that best corresponds to his/her current situation regarding the risk of developing the disease or its progression. This assessment is important for the development of a specific treatment plan or preventive strategy for that patient.

The diagnosis process may be divided into three main aspects: assessment of the risk of caries, detection of lesions, and diagnosis of caries activity.

Due to the fact that tooth decay is biofilm-sugar dependent, these are risk factors that must be evaluated in all patients, including the quality and frequency of oral hygiene, correct use of fluoride toothpaste, amount and frequency of sugar intake, dietary habits, presence of biofilm on the tooth surface, socioeconomic factors, among others [2]. A very important risk factor is that past experience of decay in children over 5 years old is undeniably the greatest risk factor for the disease [4].

The detection of carious lesions is based on a visual-tactile examination, that is, the combination of visual inspection aided by probing the dental surfaces. Other technological devices may also be included in this phase of the clinical exam, but visual-tactile examination is still the most widely used technique around the world. It is an easy, affordable, and quick method that allows the assessment of the caries lesions as well as their activity, without causing discomfort to the patient.

The dental examination should be accomplished on dental surfaces that are dry, clean, well-lit, and free from biofilm; therefore, it requires dental prophylaxis before the exam. The use of systems for detecting caries lesions, like the International Caries Detection and Assessment System (ICDAS), is advisable to standardize the examinations.

After detecting the presence of carious lesions, it is fundamental to determine their activity, that is, determining if the disease is progressing or has been inactivated. Active enamel lesions present as opaque, rough, and porous white spots. Inactive lesions already have a smooth, shiny, and polished clinical appearance. The dark color of caries lesions may be an indicative factor of inactive lesions, but it cannot be used as the sole method and evaluation factor.

The assessment of carious risk and the activity of the disease will guide the choice of different therapeutic approaches for each patient.

4. Treatment/control

The principles of Minimally Invasive Dentistry (MID) must be adopted in this phase of the treatment. Noninvasive and microinvasive techniques are the main choice to treat and control dental caries. Remineralizing strategies are fundamental during the first phases of the treatment. Patients must have sessions to educate and motivate them in order to obtain and keep good oral health, encouraging self-care capacity through access to information, skill development, and motivation. Restorative treatment should be performed aiming to favor biofilm control first, being function and esthetics as secondary objectives. Also, a restorative technique must preserve as much healthy and remineralizable tissue as possible and achieve a perfect seal while maintaining pulp and restoration integrity. Follow-up consultations must be scheduled according to the patient's needs [5]; in these consultations, all the criteria cited above must be considered again. The patient's condition will be re-evaluated and the strategies to control the disease will be reviewed, allowing for adjustments at the appropriate time.

Treatment and control of dental caries go beyond the removal of carious tissue and sealing of lesions; it is necessary to understand the etiological factors surrounding the patient to take a step forward toward solving this public health problem that affects the whole world to a greater or lesser extent.

5. Conclusion

The evolution of scientific knowledge in cariology has allowed for a paradigm shift regarding the management of dental caries. Purely surgical dental approaches focused on the elimination of cavities have been replaced by the Minimally Invasive Dentistry (MID) approach, which prioritizes prevention, remineralization, patient's education, and individualized treatment plans.

MID techniques focus on the preservation of healthy tooth structure while addressing carious lesions, aligning with the concept of early intervention to halt disease progression. By emphasizing risk assessment and individualized treatment plans, dentists can proactively manage caries risk factors. Embracing MID principles not only minimizes unnecessary tissue removal and preserves natural dentition but also promotes patient-centered care, emphasizing prevention and early intervention to mitigate the burden of dental caries effectively.

Author details

Ana Cláudia Rodrigues Chibinski
State University of Ponta Grossa, Paraná, Brazil

*Address all correspondence to: anachibinski@hotmail.com

References

[1] Qin X et al. Changes in the global burden of untreated dental caries from 1990 to 2019: A systematic analysis for the global burden of disease study. Heliyon. 2022;**8**(9):e10714

[2] Policy on social determinants of Children's Oral health and health disparities. Pediatric Dentistry. 15 Sep 2017;**39**(6):23-26. PMID: 29179307

[3] Machiulskiene V et al. Terminology of dental caries and dental caries management: Consensus report of a workshop organized by ORCA and Cariology research group of IADR. Caries Research. 2020;**54**(1):7-14

[4] Van Loveren C. Sugar restriction for caries prevention: Amount and frequency. Which is more important? Caries Research. 2019;**53**(2):168-175

[5] Wambier DS et al. Minimum intervention oral care management of early childhood caries: A 17-year follow-up case report. European Journal of Paediatric Dentistry. 2023;**24**(1):20-29

Section 2

Essays on Dental Caries

Chapter 2

Different Modalities in Caries Detection and Diagnosis

Anfal Muhammad Alqussier

Abstract

Dental caries is the most common chronic disease affecting humans worldwide. Early diagnosis of dental caries lesions allows more conservative treatment options to be followed. This may positively affect the prognosis of the condition and longevity of dental restorations. The optimum diagnosis approach should be used for better management of caries lesions. This chapter discusses several caries diagnostic modalities and systems, such as visual-tactile examination, dental radiography, transillumination-based devices, electronic caries monitors, fluorescence-based devices, and others. Furthermore, different diagnostic approaches for detecting caries lesions around different dental restorations are reviewed at the end of this chapter. Proper selection and manipulation of diagnostic tools help to enhance the outcome of dental examination. Examination should be done in clean and dry teeth for proper examination.

Keywords: dental caries/diagnosis, sensitivity and specificity, lasers*, humans, luminescent measurements/instrumentation*, cone-beam computed tomography, dental caries/diagnostic imaging, radiography, bitewing, tomography, optical coherence, ultrasonography, transillumination, fluorescence, composite resin

1. Introduction

Dental caries is a complex, noncommunicable, dynamic disease caused by biofilms. Biological, behavioral, psychological, and environmental factors all have a role in its development [1]. It has a very high incidence and prevalence throughout the world [2, 3].

The lytic effect caused by bacterial (mostly *Streptococcus mutans*) metabolism byproduct on enamel and exposed dentin surfaces is considered the main etiological factor that is responsible for enamel/dentin demineralization and breakdown [1, 3, 4]. Fortunately, dental caries is considered the most preventable disease that can be treated noninvasively when detected early [5]. Caries activity is a term that describes the mineral balance through time as net mineral loss (demineralization), net mineral gain (remineralization), or stability. Caries inactive indicates caries arrest or regression; caries active indicates caries initiation or progression [1].

Caries diagnosis is the clinical judgment to evaluate the existence of the disease by integrating relevant information, including the detection and assessment of caries signs and symptoms. In contrast, caries detection is the identification of these signs and symptoms. The primary purpose of caries diagnosis is to provide the greatest possible health outcome for the patient by enabling the selection of the most appropriate management and monitoring measures for the condition. This could be achieved by using valid and reliable detection tool/tools [1, 6]. Various caries diagnostic modalities and systems are discussed in this chapter, including visual-tactile examination, radiography, transillumination- and fluorescence-based devices, and others. Furthermore, at the end of this chapter, alternative diagnostic techniques for detecting secondary caries lesions are reviewed.

2. Diagnostic tool in caries detection

2.1 Visual-tactile examination

Although there are many different methods for caries detection, visual-tactile examination is considered the standard and the most used method in routine clinical examinations. It is usually combined with intraoral bitewing radiographs. The visual examination facilitated using a dental mirror and a ball-ended explorer should be performed gently on clean and dry teeth [5, 6]. International Caries Detection and Assessment System (ICDAS) and Nyvad Criteria are the most used scoring systems. They are used to clinically diagnose and evaluate caries based on a visual-tactile assessment [7].

Caries detection according to the visual-tactile examination method depends on the visual appearance and surface characteristic of the lesion [2, 5, 6]. Surface characteristics of the lesion may change according to the status of the caries activity. In the case of active caries lesions, the demineralization process progresses, and it is accompanied by rapid mineral loss. Active enamel caries typically appear whitish or yellowish with a loss of luster, and the texture feels soft when probed. It is frequently found in the pit and fissure, the gingival margin, and beneath the proximal contact points of both anterior and posterior teeth. They are usually covered with plaque. Moreover, active dentin lesions frequently appear brownish in color. The surface of the lesion feels soft, cheese-like, and fragile when probing [2].

On the other hand, when the demineralization process stops, the lesion is called arrested caries. The lesions' appearance is affected by the interruption of mineral loss and/or mineral regain (remineralization). The surfaces of arrested enamel lesions are often whitish or brownish in color. They are smooth and feel hard on probing. While arrested, dentin lesions frequently have dark brown/black surfaces that are hard and leathery on probing. Usually, arrested lesions are not covered with plaque [2].

Visual-tactile examination is thought to be conducted and interpreted rapidly with minimal invasion and little cost aside from professional training [5]. In addition to the excellent accuracy and diagnostic performance of the visual-tactile examination in detecting caries lesions, it allows better inspection of the interested field such as the detection of the presence of plaque accumulation which may affect the treatment planning [8]. However, relying solely on visual-tactile evaluation may lead to misdiagnoses and underestimation of early caries lesions. This occurs mostly on inaccessible surfaces, such as the proximal surfaces where adjacent teeth are present [5, 6]. To overcome its limitations, different diagnostic modalities should be allocated for caries detection in addition to visual-tactile examination during examination [8].

2.2 Intraoral bitewing radiograph

Intraoral radiographs are routinely used in conjunction with visual-tactile examination to detect caries in inaccessible areas. Bitewing radiograph is the most often utilized intraoral radiograph for evaluating inaccessible surfaces [8, 9]. It has been reported that radiograph examination is more sensitive than visual-tactile examination for detecting proximal and occlusal dentin lesions, determining lesion depth, and tracking lesion behavior [6]. The usage of intraoral digital radiography technology provides the benefit of quicker examination and image manipulation than the film radiograph technique. It allows the manipulation of image characteristics (such as contrast, brightness, sharpness, and other parameters) to improve images' clarity for better diagnosis and monitoring [5, 9].

Radiographic examination, on the other hand, has several limitations, such as exposure to ionization radiation. This might be a small but real risk, so a careful assessment of the patient's age, caries risk, and time since the last radiographs should be weighed [5]. Furthermore, radiography cannot differentiate between active and arrested lesions and occasionally between non-cavitated and cavitated lesions [6]. The performance of the examination depends on the skill and experience of the examiner, viewing conditions, and the type of the examined object [10].

In addition, intraoral radiograph radiographic examination, in conjunction with the visual-tactile examination, provides high specificity but low sensitivity in the detection of early caries lesions [5, 11]. An intraoral radiograph can detect caries lesions with only 30–60% demineralization, so it usually underestimates the extent of the caries lesions [12]. Radiographs are used in earlier diagnoses of proximal caries compared to the visual-tactile method. However, an occlusal lesion observed on a bitewing radiograph may have progressed to the middle third of the dentine. Therefore, it is no longer considered an early lesion that could be treated with remineralization techniques. This is explained by the anatomical noise caused by the complexity of superimposed crown structures on the two-dimensional images, making it harder to detect early occlusal lesions [8, 9, 12].

2.3 Cone beam computed tomography (CBCT)

Cone beam computed tomography (CBCT) is a modified type of medical computed tomography that uses a cone-beam of radiation rather than the conventional fan beam. The main advantage of the CBCT is that it provides three-dimensional (3-D) images that allow better observation and evaluation of target tissues. Furthermore, CBCT generates images in lesser radiation doses and at a lower cost than conventional medical computed tomography [11]. Several studies were conducted to evaluate the performance of CBCT in the detection of enamel and dentin caries lesions. They concluded that CBCT could be used as a valuable tool in proximal caries detection [12–14].

Compared to intraoral radiography, CBCT showed higher sensitivity in both enamel and dentin caries detection. Since the CBCT can detect caries at a lower rate of demineralization (**Figure 1**) [12–14], aside from its ease of use, the CBCT produces 3D images that are free of distortion and superimposition. Also, the images could be examined in different sections and planes, which could provide additional useful information [12].

Nonetheless, the CBCT is not widely available, which restricts its use in routine dental examinations [13]. Furthermore, because the CBCT emits more radiation than

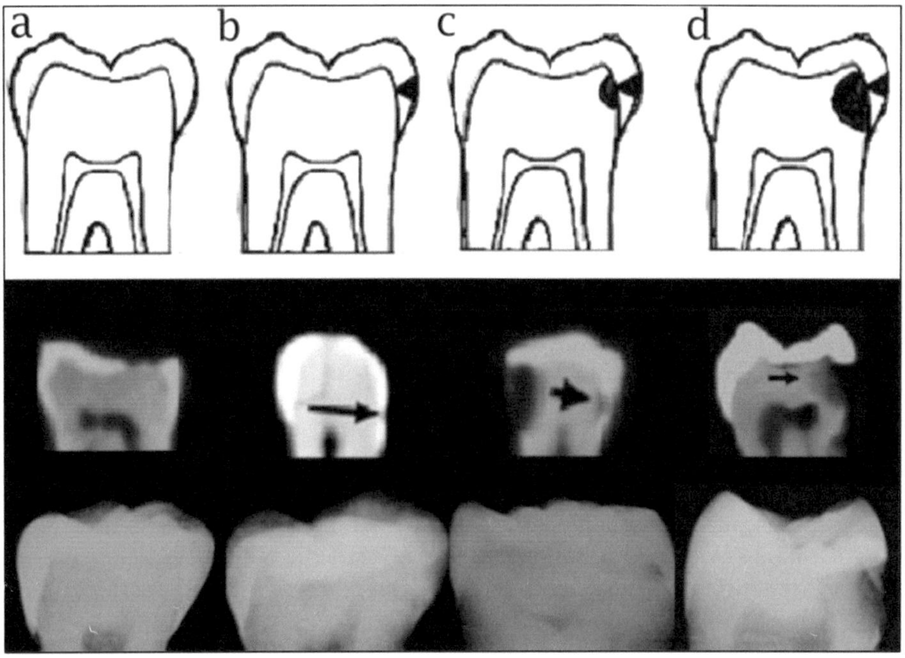

Figure 1.
Comparison of the diagnostic accuracy of CBCT and intraoral radiography for proximal caries detection. Schematic (the upper row), CBCT images (the middle row), and intraoral radiograph images (the lower row); (a) absence of proximal caries (score 0), (b) enamel caries (score 1), (c) caries extended to the outer half of dentin (score 2), and (d) caries extended to the inner half of dentin (score 3). Taken from: [12].

intraoral radiography, it is not recommended for regular caries detection. It might, however, be utilized to detect caries lesions when CBCT is used for other purposes, such as preparing for dental implant placement [12, 13].

2.4 Illumination-based devices

Other approaches for detecting caries lesions include illumination-based devices. Three types of illumination-based devices use various ways of application and interpretation: optical coherence tomography (OCT), near-infrared (NIR), and fiber-optic technology (and more recently, digital fiber optics [FOTI/DIFOTI]). Each illumination-based approach employs a distinct wavelength [5]. In the following sections, a brief discussion of each type will be issued.

2.4.1 Fiber-optic transillumination (FOTI) and digital imaging fiber-optic transillumination (DIFOTI)

Fiber-optic transillumination (FOTI) is a simple noninvasive procedure that depends on illuminating the teeth – using a hand-held device – with a high-intensity narrow beam of white light. It is considered a valid and widely accepted method for proximal caries lesion detection. Based on the principle of FOTI, a dark shadow appears when the surface with disrupted enamel crystals – due to the demineralization process – is examined. This happens due to the changes in light scattering and absorption of light photons [5, 11].

Digital imaging fiber-optic transillumination (DIFOTI) is an improvement on traditional FOTI. It works on the same principle as the FOTI and employs visible light (450–700 nm) in conjunction with a camera equipped with a charge-coupled device (CCD) that may be connected to software. DIFOTI can capture real-time images of the occlusal, buccal, and lingual surfaces. Still, a subjective interpretation of the obtained images by an examiner is required. The obtained images could be used as a reference for further monitoring of the lesion [5, 10, 11].

Fiber-optic transillumination (FOTI) is widely available in dental clinics and is easy to use. FOTI – in conjunction with visual-tactile examination – may enhance the detection of enamel proximal caries in the anterior teeth and dentin proximal caries in the posterior teeth [5]. Furthermore, DIFOTI has several advantages over bitewing radiography, including the elimination of the radiation risk associated with bitewing radiography technique, real-time image viewing, reduced patient discomfort due to the absence of intraoral films or sensors, and a higher sensitivity for early caries detection [11]. DIFOTI – in conjunction with visual-tactile examinations – is suitable for the detection of non-cavitated proximal caries. Its performance improves when the probe is placed on the buccal and lingual surfaces rather than on the occlusal surface alone [15]. An in-vitro study reported greater diagnostic accuracy of DIFOTI in the detection of proximal enamel caries in premolar teeth compared to conventional

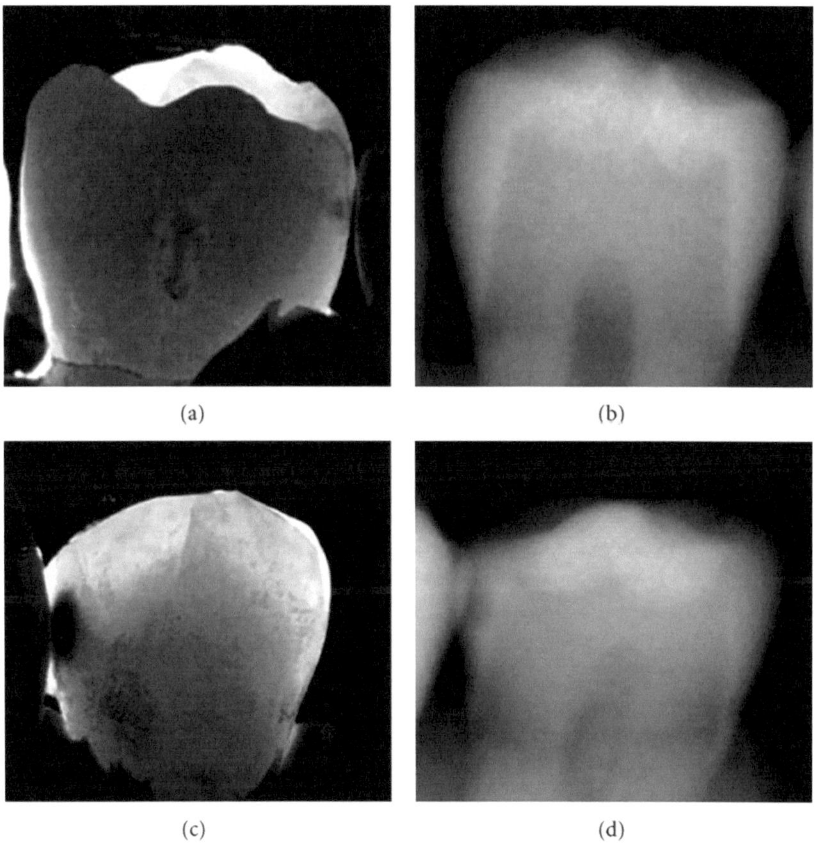

Figure 2.
Two sets of images representing enamel proximal caries using (a) DIFOTI, and (b) digital radiograph, and dentin proximal caries using (c) DIFOTI, and (b) digital radiograph. Taken from: [10].

film and digital radiographs. However, the diagnostic accuracies of the three methods in the detection of proximal dentin caries are comparable (**Figure 2**) [10].

Digital imaging fiber-optic transillumination (DIFOTI) has not been shown to objectively quantify lesion size, depth, volume, and mineral content. DIFOTI is unable to distinguish between carious lesions and developmental defects such as fluorosis. Thus, it may give high false-positive values, potentially leading to overtreatment. Furthermore, it does not determine the status of caries activity. More in-vitro and clinical studies are required to ensure and enhance the performance, diagnostic accuracy, and reliability of FOTI/DIFOTI [5, 11].

2.4.2 Near-infrared transillumination (NIRT) and near-infrared reflection (NIRR)

Near-infrared transillumination (NIRT) devices are devices that were first introduced in 2012. They use the same principle of transillumination as FOTI and DIFOTI. However, instead of visible light, these devices illuminate the tooth with near-infrared (wavelength: 780–850 nm) light with deeper penetration through the tooth structure [5, 16, 17]. The system involves a CCD sensor to obtain the images, computer connection, software, and elastic arms containing the light source. The emitted near-infrared (NIR) light can be transmitted through the gingiva, alveolar bone, tooth root, and crown. The obtained image is revealed from the occlusal surface. Like the DIFOTI, the obtained images need interpretation by an examiner [5, 16].

NIRT devices are widely available in dental clinics and are easy to use. Examples of commercially available devices include DIAGNOcam (KaVo, Biberach, Germany) and the recently introduced iTero Element 5D (Align Technologies, San Jose USA) and TRIOS 4 (3Shape, Copenhagen, Denmark) with two intraoral scanning tools [5].

Near infra-red transillumination (NIRT) device is a noninvasive tool that permits the diagnosis of non-cavitated proximal caries lesions without the risk of ionizing radiation [17]. It showed higher sensitivity than a bitewing radiograph in detecting early enamel lesions [18]. Moreover, it has been reported that NIRT showed comparable performance in detecting lesions involving the dentin-enamel junction (DEJ) to bitewing radiographs and visual-tactile examinations [18, 19].

Even though NIRT revealed a good diagnostic performance in detecting occlusal caries lesions and identifying sound teeth, it tends to overestimate [19]. In addition, NIR has low sensitivity in the detection of early enamel caries lesions [5].

Another near-infrared-based technology is the use of near-infrared reflection (NIRR) in the diagnosis of caries lesions. Both NIRT and NIRR illuminate the tooth using a near-infrared light that is scattered by carious enamel. In the NIRR method, the scattered light results in a strong reflection of the light on the sensor. Accordingly, an increase in local light intensity at a carious lesion compared to the adjacent intact tissues makes caries appear brighter. However, caries lesions are seen in the NIRT method as dark shadows due to the scattering of light within the dentin. This makes the dentin act as a homogeneous light source that illuminates the whole enamel and dentin surfaces except for the caries lesions, which appear as dark shadows [17, 20].

It has been reported that NIRR showed comparable diagnostic performance to bitewing radiograph in the detection of enamel caries lesions. However, NIRR showed some limitations. It showed low sensitivity for proximal caries detection (**Figure 3**) [17, 20, 21]. In addition, teeth with opaque enamel – especially molars – makes the detection of non-cavitated proximal caries lesion impossible with NIRR [17]. It could not be used solely in the diagnosis of proximal caries lesions. Yet, more studies are still

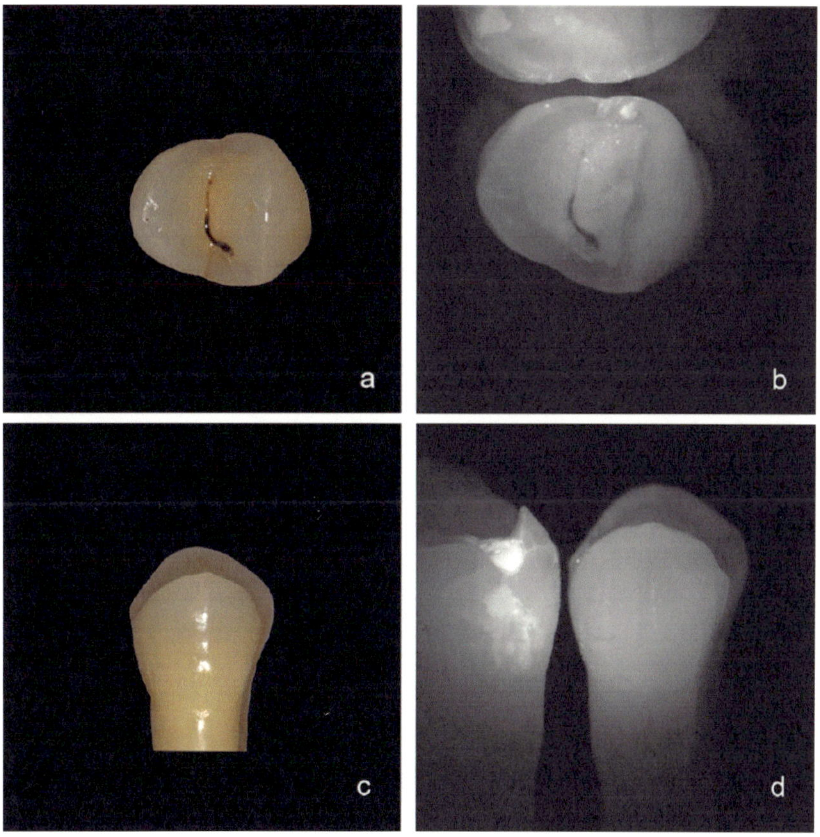

Figure 3.
Premolar with non-cavitated proximal lesion that was not detectable in clinical occlusal (a) and lingual views (c). Using NIRR, a white spot was visible in the occlusal view (b) but not in the lingual view (d). Taken from: [17].

required to evaluate and enhance the efficacy of NIRT and NIRR devices in measuring the exact lesions' depth, reliability, and validity, especially in the detection of proximal caries lesions.

2.4.3 Optical coherence tomography (OCT)

Optical coherence tomography (OCT) is an interferometric technique that establishes cross-sectional images of biological structures without the negative effect of ionization radiation exposure. It uses coherent light with a near-infrared wavelength that has maximum depth of penetration through the biological tissues [5, 7, 22]. The first use of OCT in dental research was done by Colston et al. in 1998 [23]. In dentistry, OCT is used for many applications such as caries detection, evaluation of marginal integrity of tooth restoration, and tooth crack diagnosis [11].

Optical coherence tomography (OCT) is a noninvasive tool that creates real-time 3D images at micrometer resolution through light reflection and backscattering based on the optical absorption and scattering properties of the examined tissue [7, 11]. The OCT imaging depth is significantly impacted by the medium's translucency. Structures that do not transmit light and deeper structures are irrelevant for OCT imaging. Sound enamel is practically transparent at the OCT wavelength range. The dentin-enamel junction (DEJ), which appears as a dark border, helps to distinguish between enamel and dentin in the OCT images. The caries tissues are shown as bright areas due to the development of multiple micro-porosities where the OCT signal's backscatter increases [22].

Optical coherence tomography (OCT) is an industry-ready technology that is relatively easy to use and can be applied with low optical power [24]. Compared to NIRT and FOTI devices, OCT showed superior sensitivity and better performance during caries detection. It could be used as a complementary tool with conventional clinical examination methods for clearer diagnosis [5, 7].

Swept-source optical coherence tomography (SS-OCT) is a modification type of conventional OCT systems [11, 22]. SS-OCT utilizes an interferometer with a narrow linewidth, frequency-sweep laser, and detectors to determine interference versus time. The latest SS-OCT devices provide real-time cross-sectional images with microscopic-level resolution (**Figure 4**) [22]. SS-OCT showed higher sensitivity and specificity than bitewing radiograph in caries detection at enamel and outer one-third dentin. However, for deep caries, SS-OCT showed lower sensitivity than bitewing radiograph but with similar specificity for both methods. This was explained by the greater light scattering in dentin than in enamel [25].

On the other hand, the OCT's primary flaw is the significant scattering of light at near-infrared wavelengths. Depending on the structure, this restricts the penetration depth from a few tens to hundreds of microns [24]. Furthermore, in the OCT images, the pulp chamber may not be clearly shown, thus preventing the determination of

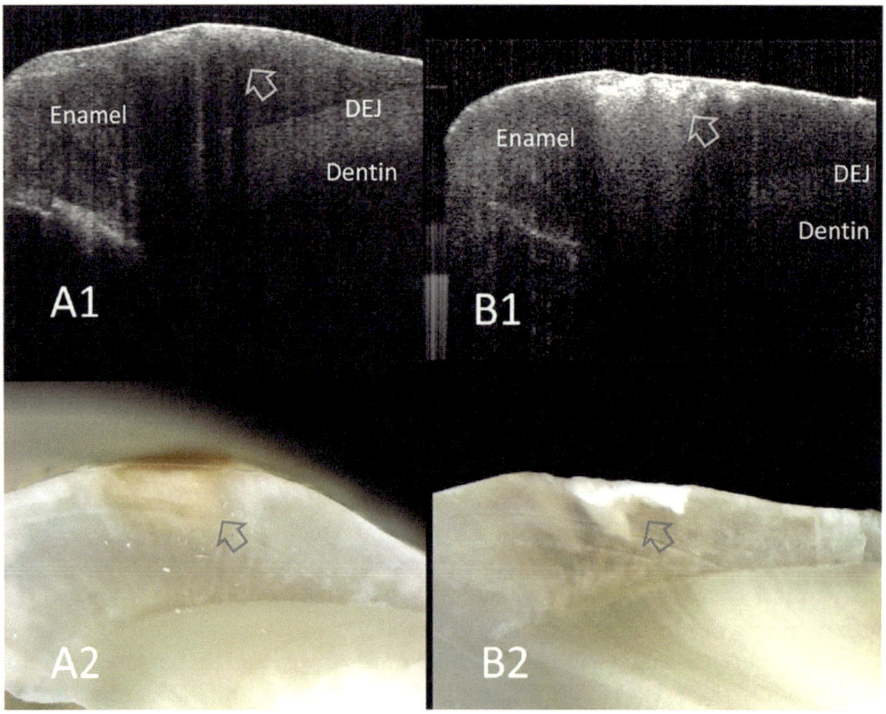

Figure 4.
SS-OCT image of smooth surface enamel caries as bright zone (white arrows) in (A1, and B1), and its corresponding histological view after cross-sectioning (A2, and B2). A non-cavitated enamel lesion is seen in (A1 and A2). However, (B1 and B2) shows a cavitated enamel lesion. Taken from: [22].

exact lesion extension concerning the pulp [25]. OCT is a noninvasive and safe method for the diagnosis of dental caries and is suitable for use in both pregnant women and small children [22]. The limited utilization of OCT devices in dental clinics is a result of their limited availability compared to OFTI and NIRT devices [5]. More studies are needed to evaluate the caries diagnostic accuracy of OCT and SS-OCT.

2.5 Electronic caries monitor (ECM)

The demineralization reaction has been shown to impact the electrical conductivity of the tooth. The bulk resistance of dental tissue is measured using the ECM device. Higher conductivity has been documented in caries teeth due to increased porosity within caries tooth structure and the presence of saliva within these pores. These result in a reduction of electrical resistance [5].

Electronic caries monitor (ECM) measures the electrical bulk resistance of dental tissue using a single, fixed-frequency alternating current. Both enamel and exposed dentin surfaces can be measured. A probe is used to send electricity through the tooth and body to a counter-electrode, which is typically kept in the patient's hand. Because the body has low resistance in comparison to dental tissues, the resistance value typically closely represents that of the tooth near the probe contact point (**Figure 5**) [26]. It has been reported that ECM is a sensitive, practical caries diagnostic tool and has been widely used in clinical studies. Utilizing ECM offers an advantage over the sole visual-tactile examination in the diagnosis of initial caries lesions diagnosis. Therefore, it has been suggested to use it in conjunction with the visual-tactile examination during dental examination [5, 26].

Although ECM is claimed to be more effective than FOTI and intraoral radiography in detecting early caries lesions, it has some limitations. As a confounding factor, the presence of stains on the investigated surfaces has been shown to affect the outcome of the ECM examination. Furthermore, the reproducibility of ECM is questionable due to the possibility of probe contact site inconsistency [5]. As a result,

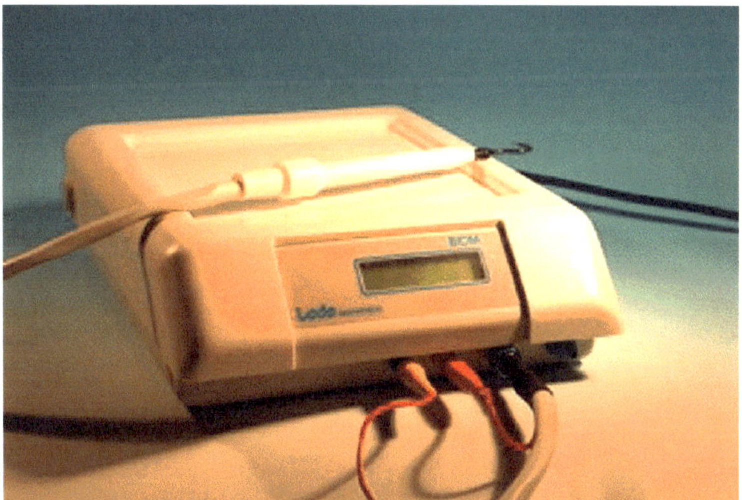

Figure 5.
Electrical caries monitor. Taken from: [26].

employing ECM to identify caries lesions should be done with caution and in combination with other caries detection methods.

2.6 Fluorescence-based devices

Demineralization of the enamel tissue results in modification of the structure's features and physical properties. Thus, If the demineralized structure is exposed to fluorescent light, it gives a different response than healthy structures. This may help in the detection and diagnosis of caries lesions. Fluorescence-based devices are classified into two categories based on the type of type of emitted light, i.e., light fluorescence, and laser fluorescence [5]. In the following sections, a brief review of each type will be discussed.

2.6.1 Light fluorescence

The qualitative light-induced fluorescence (QLF) technique can quantify small alterations in teeth based on autofluorescence, which occurs when the tooth is exposed to 405 nm visible blue light. The QLF device is composed of a light-emitted diode (LED), an inductor filter, and a metal oxide semiconductor sensor [27].

Fluorescence loss occurs because of tooth demineralization. The greater the mineral loss, the greater the loss of tooth fluorescence. Even early lesions with minor mineral changes can be detected and monitored effectively [6, 27]. When a lesion exists, an increase in light scattering causes the lesion to appear as dark patches on a bright green background. The fluorescent images of the tooth are digitalized and quantitatively assessed concerning the adjacent healthy tooth structures. A lesion is defined as any region with a reduction in fluorescence of more than 5% [6].

Qualitative light-induced fluorescence (QLF) is a noninvasive that can be used – in conjunction with the conventional visual-tactile and radiographical examination- to enhance the diagnosis of early enamel caries. It aids in the detection, quantification, and monitoring of early caries lesions that conventional methods may miss [6, 27]. Furthermore, QLF may determine both the depth and the bacterial activity of dental caries at the same time. QLF also avoids the negative consequences of radiation exposure that are linked with traditional radiographic evaluation [28].

QLF shows excellent performance and sensitivity in the detection and quantification of early smooth and occlusal caries lesions (**Figure 6**) [6]. In addition, Oh et al. reported a higher performance of QLF in the detection of occlusal caries lesions than the conventional methods alone but not in the detection of proximal caries. Because the intensity of light transmitted through the occlusal surface is already reflected before reaching the lesion in proximal caries, identification of the lesion is difficult if the degree of caries does not exceed a particular threshold [29]. The performance of the QLF evaluation may be affected by the presence of confounding factors such as the presence of dental plaque, staining, debris, and saliva [6, 29, 30]. Therefore, a clinician should not rely solely on QLF in the detection of caries lesions.

2.6.2 Laser fluorescence

Laser fluorescence (LF) is a noninvasive device used to detect caries lesions and estimate their depth by exposing the tooth to a non-ionizing laser [31]. It consists of a tip that emits monochromatic red light at 655 nm wavelength and a sensor to detect the backscattered fluorescence from the examined tooth and produce a two-dimensional hyperspectral image (**Figure 7**) [6, 31].

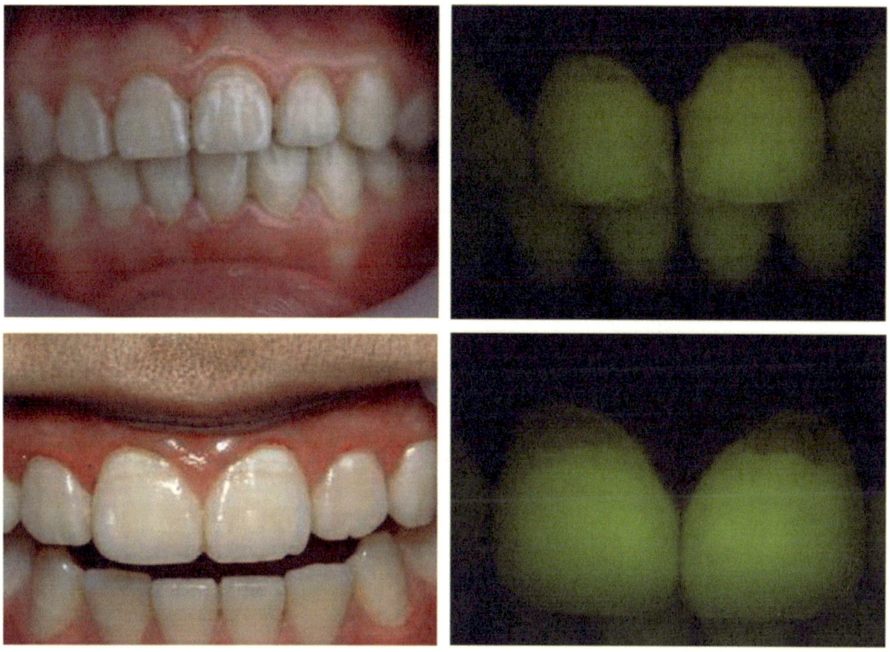

Figure 6.
Smooth surface caries detection using QLF technology. Taken from: [6].

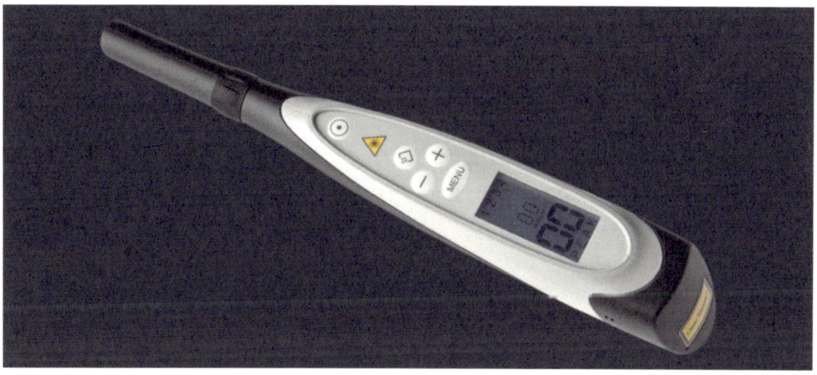

Figure 7.
Laser fluorescence caries detector (DIAGNOdent TM Pen, KaVo). Taken from: https://www.kavo.com.

Carious teeth generate fluorescence proportional to the degree of caries, whereas clean and healthy teeth produce no or little fluorescence. It was proposed that these fluorescence changes are caused by protoporphyrin, a photosensitive pigment found in carious tissues as a consequence of bacterial metabolic activity [11].

Laser fluorescence (LF) has been found to tend to higher specificity than sensitivity for enamel caries detection. The performance of the LF is better with larger lesions [6]. In addition, Kapor et al. concluded that LF examination shows high sensitivity and specificity. However, it should not be used alone to avoid overtreatment [8]. In comparison to QLF, Diniz et al. reported higher sensitivity of laser fluorescence device (LF pen) in the detection of occlusal caries [32].

Several confounding factors, including the amount of plaque, calculus, and/or discoloration on the tooth surface, as well as the degree of dehydration of dental tissue, may influence the LF evaluation [6]. Thus, LF may be used as an adjunct examination method to enhance the detection of early caries lesions that could not be detected properly using visual-tactile examination alone.

2.7 Frequency-domain infrared photothermal radiometry and modulated luminescence (PTR/LUM)

Photothermal radiometry and modulated luminescence PTR/LUM technology are based on the detection of optical and thermal changes in the tooth structure [33]. PTR is based on the modulated thermal infrared response (also known as a black body or plank radiation) of a medium because of repeatedly exposing a specimen to radiation. Black body radiation is the electromagnetic energy emitted by a black body when its temperature is constant and uniform, or from a body that is in thermodynamic equilibrium with its surroundings. The sample surface's temperature changes because of the absorbed radiation energy being transformed into thermal energy. A PTR signal-generating infrared detector can be used to measure the change in thermal emissions due to temperature modulation. LUM depends on the transformation of optical energy into radiation energy. When optical energy from a laser source is absorbed by a molecule, it causes excitement to its chromophores into a higher energy status. Then, after de-excitation to lower energy status, longer wavelength energy will be emitted. This could be detected by a photodetector that generates a LUM signal [34].

Canary caries detection system is based on PTR/LUM technology [11]. It was developed by Quantum Dental Technologies (Toronto, ON, Canada) in 2009 and used in a Health Canada-approved human investigational trial [34]. According to the manufacturer, the Canary caries detection system (**Figure 8**) can detect caries from 50 to 5 mm depth including secondary caries detection around sealant and restorations' margins. Canary caries detection system values are not affected by stains and the presence of calculus or saliva [11].

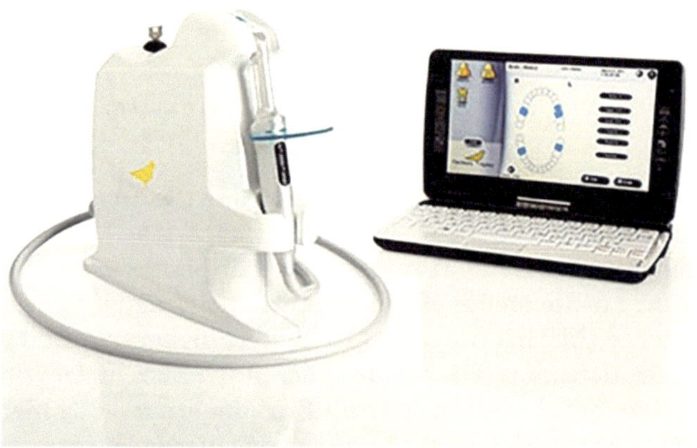

Figure 8.
The canary system from quantum dental technologies. Taken from: https://www.dentalcompare.com.

An in-vitro study compared the performance of the Canary caries detection system in the detection of proximal caries lesions to the performance of visual-tactile and radiographical examinations. They used polarized light microscopy as a gold standard in caries detection. A higher sensitivity of the PTR/LUM caries detection system compared to the other two examinations tested was reported. There was no significant difference in specificity between the radiographical examination and the PTR/LUM method. In contrast, the specificity of the visual-tactile examination was the lowest among the three examination methods [33]. In addition, a study by Xing et al., in 2023, reported a positive moderate correlation with the caries depth of the PTR/LUM system; even a 20° deviation from perpendicular did not affect its performance [35]. Also, it has been reported that the PTR/LUM system can detect non-cavitied proximal lesions without the use of ionization radiation [36]. However, the PTR/LUM caries detection method is still considered new, and more in-vitro and clinical studies are required to evaluate its performance and accuracy.

2.8 Ultrasound

The first use of ultrasound in dentistry was by Baum et al. in 1963 [37]. Sound waves with frequencies (20 kHz) higher than those heard by humans are used in ultrasound technology. During caries detection, ultrasound depends on the substantial variations in sonic conductivity between sound and demineralized dental structures. The use of ultrasound to detect caries is considered simple, safe, and provides real-time images, among other benefits [11]. A recent study reported a high correlation between histological and ultrasound examinations' results in the detection of smooth surface enamel caries [38].

Although it showed promising performance in caries detection, there are only limited studies done to evaluate the efficacy of the ultrasound system for caries detection.

3. Detection of secondary caries lesions

Secondary caries (also known as recurrent caries) are caries lesions that form near the margin of a restoration. Other examination approaches besides the visual-tactile assessment could improve the longevity of the restoration. Secondary caries could be predicted by the presence of marginal ditching, discoloration of adjacent tooth structures, and gaps at the tooth-restoration interface. Unfortunately, these signs are not reliable predictors making the detection of secondary caries lesions with solely visual examination challenging. Alternatively, relying solely on radiographic evaluation may result in an underestimate of lesion extent. The radiopacity of restorative materials may contribute to secondary caries misdiagnosis [39].

Several studies suggested the use of LF along with visual-tactile and radiographical examinations for the detection of secondary lesions [40, 41]. While NIR transillumination appears to be promising in the detection of secondary caries, there is little data to support it. Even though just a few studies have been conducted to evaluate the use of visual-tactile evaluation with QLF, this method has demonstrated poor performance [40].

While CBCT images detect proximal caries more correctly than bitewing radiography, the presence of high-density restorative materials such as dental amalgam and porcelain restorations results in metal artifacts. This lowers the CBCT's

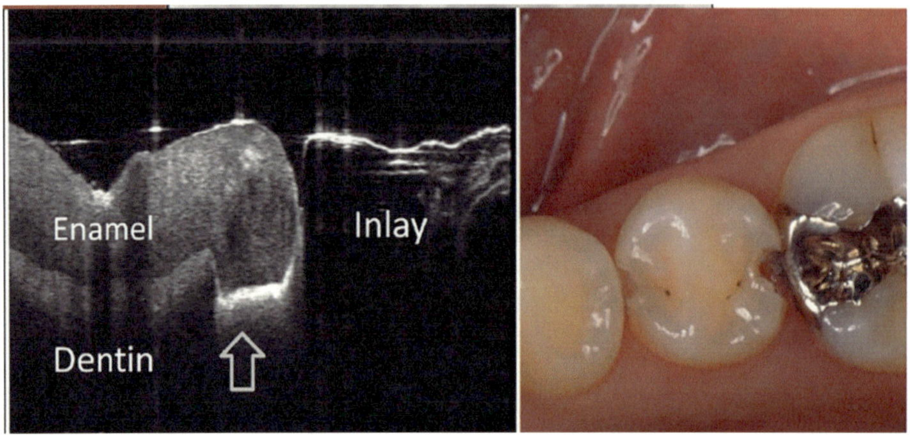

Figure 9.
SS-OCT is not able to detect caries lesion underneath the metal alloy in the first molar. SS-OCT image of proximal contacts between second premolar and first molar (scanning from occlusal surface). A distinct white line indicates the presence of caries (arrow). Cross-sectional imaging of the first molar is not possible due to the metal inlay (right). The presence of dentin caries in the mesial and distal proximal surfaces of the second premolar is confirmed after cavity preparation (left). Taken from: [22].

accuracy in detecting secondary caries lesions. Because of its atomic number and density, amalgam restoration produces more artifacts than porcelain and metal-ceramic restoration. As a result, there are more false-positive results [12]. However, other studies showed higher diagnostic accuracy of CBCT compared to bitewing radiography in the detection of secondary caries around resin composite restorations [14, 42].

Optical coherence tomography (OCT) has also been investigated for the detection of secondary caries. The presence of opaque and metallic restoration makes subsequent caries detection with OCT challenging (**Figure 9**). However, the satisfactory performance of the OCT in detecting secondary caries around tooth-colored restorations that can transmit light has been documented [22]. In addition, the detection of secondary caries around tooth-colored restorations could be established by the PTR/LUM system. Abrams et al. reported that the PTR/LUM system (The Canary System, CS) has the potential for more accurate diagnosis of secondary caries around compomer and resin-modified glass ionomer restorations than visual-tactile examination, light-emitting diodes fluorescence, and LF used [43].

Based on the exceeding, adjunctive diagnostic aids – in addition to conventional visual-tactile and radiographic examinations – should be used when detecting secondary caries lesions to improve diagnostic outcomes and avoid overtreatment. This is particularly applied when examining teeth with high-opacity restorations. Restorations' finishing may be required to overcome the limits of some diagnostic aids that are influenced by the presence of staining.

4. Conclusion

In conclusion, the most common and widely used approach for caries detection and assessment is a visual-tactile examination combined with a radiographic examination. It does, however, have certain limits. As a result, various diagnostic tools and modalities are available and might be employed to improve caries diagnosis accuracy and sensitivity. A proper caries detection method should be carefully selected and implemented on clean and dry surfaces. More laboratory and clinical research is required to assess and improve the performance of such methods.

Conflict of interest

The author declares no conflict of interest.

Author details

Anfal Muhammad Alqussier
Restorative Dental Science Department, College of Dentistry, Taibah University, Al-Madinah al-Munawwarah, Saudi Arabia

*Address all correspondence to: anfal.m.q@gmail.com

References

[1] MacHiulskiene V, Campus G, Carvalho JC, Dige I, Ekstrand KR, Jablonski-Momeni A, et al. Terminology of dental caries and dental caries management: Consensus report of a workshop organized by ORCA and Cariology Research Group of IADR. Caries Research. 2020;**54**(1):7-14. DOI: 10.1159/000503309

[2] Cheng L, Zhang L, Yue L, Ling J, Fan M, Yang D, et al. Expert consensus on dental caries management. International Journal of Oral Science. 2022;**14**(1):13-17. DOI: 10.1038/S41368-022-00167-3

[3] Pitts NB, Twetman S, Fisher J, Marsh PD. Understanding dental caries as a non-communicable disease. British Dental Journal. 2021;**231**(12):749-753. DOI: 10.1038/S41415-021-3775-4

[4] Lemos JA, Palmer SR, Zeng L, Wen ZT, Kajfasz JK, Freires IA, et al. The biology of Streptococcus mutans. Microbiology Spectrum. 2019;**7**(1): GPP3-0051-2018. DOI: 10.1128/MICROBIOLSPEC.GPP3-0051-2018

[5] Macey R, Walsh T, Riley P, Hogan R, Glenny AM, Worthington HV, et al. Transillumination and optical coherence tomography for the detection and diagnosis of enamel caries. Cochrane Database of Systematic Reviews. 2021;**1**(1):CD013855. DOI: 10.1002/14651858.CD013855

[6] Gomez J. Detection and diagnosis of the early caries lesion. BMC Oral Health. 2015;**15**(1):S3. DOI: 10.1186/1472-6831-15-S1-S3

[7] Mohamad Saberi FN, Sukumaran P, Ung NM, Liew YM. Assessment of demineralized tooth lesions using optical coherence tomography and other state-of-the-art technologies: A review. Biomedical Engineering Online. 2022;**21**(1):83. DOI: 10.1186/S12938-022-01055-X

[8] Kapor S, Rankovic MJ, Khazaei Y, Crispin A, Schüler I, Krause F, et al. Systematic review and meta-analysis of diagnostic methods for occlusal surface caries. Clinical Oral Investigations. 2021;**25**(8):4801-4815. DOI: 10.1007/S00784-021-04024-1

[9] Obuchowicz R, Nurzynska K, Obuchowicz B, Urbanik A, Piórkowski A. Caries detection enhancement using texture feature maps of intraoral radiographs. Oral Radiology. 2020;**36**(3):275-287. DOI: 10.1007/S11282-018-0354-8

[10] Ástvaldsdóttir Á, Åhlund K, Holbrook WP, De Verdier B, Tranæus S. Approximal caries detection by DIFOTI: In vitro comparison of diagnostic accuracy/efficacy with film and digital radiography. International Journal of Dentistry. 2012;**2012**:326401. DOI: 10.1155/2012/326401

[11] Abogazalah N, Ando M. Alternative methods to visual and radiographic examinations for approximal caries detection. Journal of Oral Science. 2017;**59**(3):315-322. DOI: 10.2334/JOSNUSD.16-0595

[12] Mosavat F, Ahmadi E, Amirfarhangi S, Rafeie N. Evaluation of diagnostic accuracy of CBCT and intraoral radiography for proximal caries detection in the presence of different dental restoration materials. BMC Oral Health. 2023;**23**(1):419. DOI: 10.1186/S12903-023-02954-8

[13] Walsh T, Macey R, Riley P, Glenny AM, Schwendicke F, Worthington HV,

et al. Imaging modalities to inform the detection and diagnosis of early caries. Cochrane Database of Systematic Reviews. 2021;**3**(3):CD014545. DOI: 10.1002/14651858.CD014545

[14] Kasraei S, Shokri A, Poorolajal J, Khajeh S, Rahmani H. Comparison of cone-beam computed tomography and intraoral radiography in detection of recurrent caries under composite restorations. Brazilian Dental Journal. 2017;**28**(1):85-91. DOI: 10.1590/0103-644020170124

[15] Abogazalah N, Eckert GJ, Ando M. In vitro visual and visible light transillumination methods for detection of natural non-cavitated approximal caries. Clinical Oral Investigations. 2019;**23**(3):1287-1294. DOI: 10.1007/S00784-018-2546-3

[16] Söchtig F, Hickel R, Kühnisch J. Caries detection and diagnostics with near-infrared light transillumination: Clinical experiences. Quintessence International. 2014;**45**(6):531-538. DOI: 10.3290/J.QI.A31533

[17] Heck K, Litzenburger F, Geitl T, Kunzelmann KH. Near-infrared reflection at 780 nm for detection of early proximal caries in posterior permanent teeth in vitro. Dento Maxillo Facial Radiology. 2021;**50**(6):20210005. DOI: 10.1259/DMFR.20210005

[18] Metzger Z, Colson DG, Bown P, Weihard T, Baresel I, Nolting T. Reflected near-infrared light versus bite-wing radiography for the detection of proximal caries: A multicenter prospective clinical study conducted in private practices. Journal of Dentistry. 2022;**116**:103861. DOI: 10.1016/J.JDENT.2021.103861

[19] Litzenburger F, Lederer A, Kollmuß M, Hickel R, Kunzelmann KH, Heck K. Near-infrared transillumination with high dynamic range imaging for occlusal caries detection in vitro. Lasers in Medical Science. 2020;**35**(9):2049-2058. DOI: 10.1007/S10103-020-03078-Z

[20] Lederer A, Kunzelmann KH, Heck K, Hickel R, Litzenburger F. In vitro validation of near-infrared transillumination at 780 nm for the detection of caries on proximal surfaces. Clinical Oral Investigations. 2019;**23**(11):3933-3940. DOI: 10.1007/S00784-019-02824-0

[21] Litzenburger F, Heck K, Kaisarly D, Kunzelmann KH. Diagnostic validity of early proximal caries detection using near-infrared imaging technology on 3D range data of posterior teeth. Clinical Oral Investigations. 2022;**26**(1):543-553. DOI: 10.1007/S00784-021-04032-1

[22] Shimada Y, Yoshiyama M, Tagami J, Sumi Y. Evaluation of dental caries, tooth crack, and age-related changes in tooth structure using optical coherence tomography. Japanese Dental Science Review. 2020;**56**(1):109-118. DOI: 10.1016/J.JDSR.2020.08.001

[23] Colston BW, Everett MJ, Da Silva LB, Otis LL, Stroeve P, Nathel H. Imaging of hard- and soft-tissue structure in the oral cavity by optical coherence tomography. Applied Optics. 1998;**37**(16):3582. DOI: 10.1364/AO.37.003582

[24] Israelsen NM, Petersen CR, Barh A, Jain D, Jensen M, Hannesschläger G, et al. Real-time high-resolution mid-infrared optical coherence tomography. Light: Science & Applications. 2019;**8**(1):11. DOI: 10.1038/S41377-019-0122-5

[25] Shimada Y, Nakagawa H, Sadr A, Wada I, Nakajima M, Nikaido T, et al. Noninvasive cross-sectional imaging of proximal caries using swept-source optical coherence tomography (SS-OCT) in vivo. Journal of Biophotonics. 2014;7(7):506-513. DOI: 10.1002/JBIO.201200210

[26] Pretty IA, Ellwood RP. The caries continuum: Opportunities to detect, treat and monitor the re-mineralization of early caries lesions. Journal of Dentistry. 2013;**41**(Suppl. 2):S12-S21. DOI: 10.1016/j.jdent.2010.04.003

[27] Oh SH, Choi JY, Kim SH. Evaluation of dental caries detection with quantitative light-induced fluorescence in comparison to different field of view devices. Scientific Reports. 2022;**12**(1):6139. DOI: 10.1038/s41598-022-10126-x

[28] Cho KH, Kang CM, Jung HI, Lee HS, Lee K, Lee TY, et al. The diagnostic efficacy of quantitative light-induced fluorescence in detection of dental caries of primary teeth. Journal of Dentistry. 2021;**115**:103845. DOI: 10.1016/j.jdent.2021.103845

[29] Oh SH, Lee SR, Choi JY, Choi YS, Kim SH, Yoon HC, et al. Detection of dental caries and cracks with quantitative light-induced fluorescence in comparison to radiographic and visual examination: A retrospective case study. Sensors (Basel). 2021;**21**(5):1-15. DOI: 10.3390/s21051741

[30] Amaechi BT, Higham SM. Quantitative light-induced fluorescence: A potential tool for general dental assessment. Journal of Biomedical Optics. 2002;**7**(1):7. DOI: 10.1117/1.1427044

[31] El-Sharkawy YH, Elbasuney S. Non-invasive caries detection and delineation via novel laser-induced fluorescence with hyperspectral imaging. Photodiagnosis and Photodynamic Therapy. 2022;**40**:103186. DOI: 10.1016/j.pdpdt.2022.103186

[32] Diniz MB, Campos PH, Wilde S, Cordeiro RCL, Zandona AGF. Performance of light-emitting diode device in detecting occlusal caries in the primary molars. Lasers in Medical Science. 2019;**34**(6):1235-1241. DOI: 10.1007/s10103-019-02717-4

[33] Jan J, Wan Bakar WZ, Mathews SM, Okoye LO, Ehler BR, Louden C, et al. Proximal caries lesion detection using the canary caries detection system: An in vitro study. Journal of Investigative and Clinical Dentistry. 2016;**7**(4):383-390. DOI: 10.1111/jicd.12163

[34] Garcia JA, Mandelis A, Abrams SH, Matvienko A. Photothermal radiometry and modulated luminescence: Applications for dental caries detection. In: Popp J, Tuchin VV, Chiou A, Heinemann SH, editors. Handbook of Biophotonics, Vol. 2: Photonics for Health Care. Berlin: Wiley-VCH; 2011. pp. 1047-1052

[35] Xing H, Eckert GJ, Ando M. Impact of angle on photothermal radiometry and modulated luminescence (PTR/LUM) value. Journal of Dentistry. 2023;**132**:104500. DOI: 10.1016/j.jdent.2023.104500

[36] Xing H, Eckert GJ, Ando M. Detection ability and direction effect of photothermal-radiometry and modulated-luminescence for non-cavitated approximal caries. Journal of Dentistry. 2019;**90**:103221. DOI: 10.1016/j.jdent.2019.103221

[37] Baum G, Greenwood I, Slawski S, Smirnow R. Observation of internal structures of teeth by ultrasonography. Science. 1963;**139**(3554):495-496. DOI: 10.1126/science.139.3554.495

[38] Yanikoglu F, Avci H, Celik ZC, Tagtekin D. Diagnostic performance of ICDAS II, FluoreCam and ultrasound for flat surface caries with different depths. Ultrasound in Medicine & Biology. 2020;**46**(7):1755-1760. DOI: 10.1016/j.ultrasmedbio.2020.03.007

[39] Signori C, Gimenez T, Mendes FM, Huysmans MCDNJM, Opdam NJM,

Cenci MS. Clinical relevance of studies on the visual and radiographic methods for detecting secondary caries lesions - A systematic review. Journal of Dentistry. 2018;**75**:22-33. DOI: 10.1016/j.jdent.2018.05.018

[40] Askar H, Krois J, Göstemeyer G, Bottenberg P, Zero D, Banerjee A, et al. Secondary caries: What is it, and how it can be controlled, detected, and managed? Clinical Oral Investigations. 2020;**24**(5):1869-1876. DOI: 10.1007/s00784-020-03268-7

[41] Brouwer F, Askar H, Paris S, Schwendicke F. Detecting secondary caries lesions: A systematic review and meta-analysis. Journal of Dental Research. 2016;**95**(2):143-151. DOI: 10.1177/0022034515611041

[42] Talachi F, Abesi F, Ezoji F, Mahjoub S, Ghorbani H, Bijani A. Comparison of accuracy cone-beam computed tomography and digital bitewing radiography for detection of recurrent caries under various restorative materials: In vitro study. Oral Radiology. 2023;**39**(4):722-730. DOI: 10.1007/s11282-023-00690-x

[43] Abrams T, Abrams S, Sivagurunathan K, Moravan V, Hellen W, Elman G, et al. Detection of caries around resin-modified glass ionomer and compomer restorations using four different modalities in vitro. Dentistry Journal (Basel). 2018;**6**(3):47. DOI: 10.3390/dj6030047

Chapter 3

Revolutionizing Dental Caries Diagnosis through Artificial Intelligence

Sukumaran Anil, Krishnaa Sudeep, Sudeep Saratchandran and Vishnupriya K. Sweety

Abstract

The diagnosis and management of dental caries, a prevalent global oral health issue, have traditionally depended on clinical examination and the interpretation of radiographic images. However, with the rapid advancements in technology, the landscape of dental diagnostics is transforming. This chapter delves into the revolutionary impact of artificial intelligence (AI) on detecting and managing dental caries. Dental professionals can now achieve enhanced diagnostic accuracy by harnessing the power of machine learning algorithms and image recognition technologies, even identifying early-stage caries that conventional methods might overlook. The integration of AI into dentistry not only promises improved patient outcomes by facilitating timely interventions and streamlining clinical workflows, potentially redefining the future of oral healthcare. While the prospects are promising, it is imperative to concurrently address the challenges and ethical considerations accompanying AI-driven diagnostics to ensure that the technology augments, rather than supplants, the expertise of dental professionals. The chapter serves as a comprehensive overview of the current state of AI in dental caries diagnosis, its potential benefits, and the road ahead.

Keywords: dental caries, artificial intelligence, machine learning, early diagnosis, clinical decision-making, diagnostic imaging, image interpretation

1. Introduction

Dental caries is a pervasive global oral health issue, impacting individuals across all age demographics. Recognized by the World Health Organization as a significant public health challenge, it carries a substantial health burden due to its ubiquity and potential for severe complications [1]. This chronic condition is marked by the gradual degradation of dental hard tissues, primarily due to the metabolic activities of oral bacteria [2]. Such deterioration stems from the demineralization of tooth enamel and dentine, a result of acids produced by bacteria in plaque-a sticky film that continually forms on teeth. The etiological factors underpinning dental caries are diverse, encompassing microbial presence, dietary habits, host reactions, and temporal elements [2]. While initial manifestations might be subtle lesions on the enamel, unchecked progression can lead to pronounced cavitations, threatening the tooth's structural integrity and paving the way for more grave dental issues, including pain, infection, tooth loss, and even broader systemic health complications [3].

Technology has been a driving force in improving oral healthcare, especially in recent decades. Artificial Intelligence (AI) stands out among the technologies making a transformative impact. At its core, AI is a branch of computer science that aims to create machines that mimic human intelligence [4]. This includes learning from experience, understanding language, recognizing patterns, solving problems, and making decisions. AI has many applications, from autonomous vehicles and voice assistants to healthcare diagnostics and treatment planning. AI has shown promising potential in healthcare, enhancing precision, improving patient outcomes, and streamlining processes. It has been applied in various areas, such as radiology, cardiology, oncology, and, more recently, dentistry. In the context of dental care, AI can offer several advantages. For instance, it can automate routine tasks, assist in the interpretation of radiographs, aid in diagnosing oral conditions, and even predict the risk of future oral health problems. This has profound implications for managing dental caries, where early and accurate detection is paramount. The use of AI in dentistry is an evolving field, with advancements in Machine Learning (ML), a subset of AI that uses statistical methods to enable machines to improve with experience, and image recognition playing a significant role [5]. These technologies have enabled the development of systems that can analyze dental radiographs or intraoral images, detect signs of dental caries, and alert the dentist to potential areas of concern.

However, as with any technological innovation, challenges and ethical considerations must be considered. Integrating AI into clinical practice requires understanding these aspects and strategies to manage them [6]. Despite these challenges, the potential of AI to revolutionize dental care is considerable. The promise of AI for the future of dental caries management is exciting. It can enhance accuracy in diagnosis, optimize treatment planning, improve patient outcomes, and advance dental care delivery. This chapter aims to provide a comprehensive understanding of the role of AI in dental caries, highlighting its potential, exploring its applications, discussing challenges and ethical considerations, and speculating about future directions.

2. Methods for diagnosing dental caries

Dental caries is one of the most widespread chronic diseases globally, affecting individuals across the lifespan. Effective management of dental caries hinges on early detection and accurate diagnosis [7]. Over time, several diagnostic methods have been developed and employed in dental practice, each with merits and limitations. The main techniques for diagnosing dental caries are visual-tactile examination, radiographic evaluation, and advanced imaging technologies [8].

2.1 Visual-tactile examination

The visual-tactile examination is the most basic and commonly used method for caries diagnosis. It involves thoroughly examining the teeth using a dental explorer and mirror, accompanied by sufficient lighting. The dentist assesses the teeth' color, texture, and transparency, looking for signs of decay such as discolorations, cavitations, or changes in enamel reflection. While this method is simple and cost-effective, it has limitations [8]. Early dental caries may not cause noticeable changes in the tooth's appearance, making visual-tactile examinations less effective for detecting caries in their initial stages.

2.2 Photographs

Intraoral photographs serve as valuable aids in diagnosing dental caries. High-quality digital images allow for visualizing teeth in detail, which can help identify early signs of caries. Photographs also enable longitudinal assessment of a patient's oral health, allowing for comparison over time to detect changes or progressions in dental caries [9]. However, while photographs can provide detailed surface images, they cannot provide insights into subsurface structures or the extent of internal decay.

2.3 Radiographic examination

Radiographic examinations, particularly dental bitewing X-rays, are widely used to diagnose dental caries [10]. They offer the ability to visualize both the surface and subsurface structures of teeth, enabling the detection of caries that might be hidden from the naked eye or in areas like interproximal spaces, which are hard to inspect visually. There are two primary types of dental X-rays: bitewings and periapical. Bitewing X-rays are beneficial for detecting caries in the crowns of teeth, especially between the teeth. In contrast, periapical X-rays can show the entire tooth, including the roots, and help detect abscesses and cysts [11]. However, radiation exposure, albeit minimal, and the potential for overdiagnosis are considerations with radiographic examinations.

2.4 Advanced imaging techniques

In recent years, advanced imaging techniques have emerged that aim to overcome the limitations of traditional methods. These include optical coherence tomography (OCT), laser fluorescence devices (DIAGNOdent), and near-infrared light transillumination [12]. For example, OCT can provide detailed, cross-sectional images of dental tissues, allowing for the early detection of caries. Laser fluorescence devices measure changes in tooth fluorescence to identify carious lesions. Near-infrared light transillumination exploits the different light-scattering properties of healthy and carious dental tissues to detect decay. While promising, these techniques have yet to be widely used in routine dental practice, primarily due to their cost and the need for specialized equipment and training.

Diagnosing dental caries involves a combination of methods, from the traditional visual-tactile examination to advanced imaging techniques. Each method has strengths and limitations, and the choice often depends on the clinical scenario, the dentist's expertise, and available resources [13]. As research progresses and technology advances, we can anticipate more precise and effective tools for caries detection, leading to improved patient outcomes.

3. The role of AI in dental caries diagnosis

The integration of Artificial Intelligence in healthcare has opened new avenues for enhancing patient care, and dentistry is no exception. The use of AI in dentistry has been a transformative step, promising more accurate diagnoses, more efficient practices, and better patient outcomes. The use of AI in dentistry is only partially a recent development [14]. The journey began in the late 20th century with expert systems that attempted to replicate the decision-making abilities of dental experts. For instance, the DENTSYS system developed in the 1980s used AI to generate dental treatment plans. However, in the last decade, AI's application in dentistry has gained significant momentum, spurred by advancements in machine learning algorithms and increased computing power. Researchers and tech companies developed AI tools to analyze dental images and detect oral conditions, including dental caries [15].

AI's importance in managing dental caries cannot be overstated. Dental caries is a prevalent condition, often requiring time-intensive analysis of dental images for diagnosis. AI systems, particularly those using machine learning, can quickly analyze these images and detect signs of caries. They save time and can improve the accuracy of diagnosis by catching early-stage caries that the human eye may miss [16]. AI can also be used to predict the risk of dental caries. By analyzing patient data and identifying risk factors, AI systems can predict a patient's likelihood of developing caries in the future. This allows for early intervention and preventive care, which is more cost-effective and beneficial for the patient's oral health [17].

The pressing need for early detection and intervention is evident. With the advent of digital dentistry, the incorporation of Artificial Intelligence (AI) heralds a transformative approach in the detection, management, and prophylaxis of dental caries, highlighting the significance of this condition both clinically and in the broader public health context. Artificial Intelligence (AI), an area that seeks to emulate human cognitive functions through machines, has witnessed rapid advancements over the past decades and has infiltrated various domains of healthcare, revolutionizing diagnostic and therapeutic processes [18]. Its integration within dentistry, particularly in dental caries detection and management, has shown promising potential. This chapter delves into AI's role in dental caries, offering insights into its applications, benefits, challenges, and prospects. But before we proceed to understand AI's role, it is pivotal to have a foundational understanding of dental caries. This condition remains one of the most prevalent oral diseases globally.

4. AI methods used for diagnosis of dental caries from photographs and X-rays

4.1 Reinforcement learning

This type of machine learning, where an agent learns by taking actions in an environment to optimize a reward, has seen less prominence in medical imaging than in supervised or unsupervised methods. Nevertheless, it holds substantial promise for specific applications. In dental imaging, reinforcement learning can serve vital roles, such as guiding image segmentation or pinpointing optimal imaging parameters. Ren et al. (2021) highlighted that this approach's potential in dental diagnostics is considerable [19].

4.2 Generative adversarial networks (GANs)

Generative Adversarial Networks, commonly known as GANs, are at the forefront of unsupervised machine learning algorithms, characterized by their unique structure of two contesting neural networks. These networks, working in tandem, have historically been deployed to craft synthetic images that closely replicate real ones. However, their application is not confined to this realm alone. Increasingly, GANs are finding utility in augmenting data sets, creating additional synthetic training examples, and, crucially, anomaly detection. In dentistry, for instance, they can effectively identify teeth conditions that deviate from the expected, such as dental caries [20].

4.3 Support vector machines (SVMs)

SVMs, are specialized supervised learning models tailored for classification and regression tasks. In dental imaging, SVMs play an instrumental role in classifying images, particularly in determining the presence or absence of caries [21]. The distinctive feature of SVMs lies in their ability to generate a boundary, a demarcation that effectively separates various image classes. This separation is not arbitrary; the algorithm constructs it to ensure the maximal margin between the differing image categories [22].

4.4 Random forests

Random Forests are ensemble machine-learning algorithms that build upon multiple decision trees. The output is derived from the class mode of the results produced by these individual trees. As an ensemble learning method, it amalgamates the predictions from various machine learning models to yield a more precise prediction [23]. As corroborated by Breiman, when applied to dental health, Random Forests are particularly adept at classifying dental images and even forecasting the progression of diseases such as dental caries [24].

4.5 Semantic segmentation

Semantic Segmentation is a pivotal technique in computer vision that classifies individual pixels within an image into distinct categories. Applied to dental radiographs, this method can deftly categorize pixels into labels such as 'healthy tissue,' 'caries,' or 'other.' Such granular, pixel-level analysis furnishes a comprehensive assessment of dental images, facilitating the pinpointing of the exact location and extent of dental caries, thus aiding in accurate diagnostics [25].

4.6 Self-supervised learning

Self-Supervised Learning is a nuanced approach in machine learning, distinguished by its reliance on data's inherent structure for guidance. Abandoning the conventional dependence on explicit labels, these sophisticated algorithms derive pseudo-labels from the data to discern representations. Within the realm of dental caries detection, this methodology emerges as particularly advantageous [26]. By harnessing the power of extensive unlabeled dental image datasets, self-supervised learning can amplify a model's adeptness at extracting salient features. These enhanced models, equipped to predict sequences or deduce image orientations, set the stage for monumental advancements in diagnostic precision [27].

4.7 Capsule networks

Capsule Networks, often called CapsNets, represent a pioneering stride in artificial neural networks. Their unique strength lies in capturing hierarchical relationships intrinsic to data. Traditional neural networks might overlook specific details in their processing, but CapsNets stand apart by meticulously preserving nuanced data aspects, encompassing spatial relationships and other intricate properties [28]. This retention of detail augments their potential, making them particularly favorable for specialized tasks such as dental caries detection. In such applications, understanding the spatial interplay between distinct tooth components becomes pivotal for accurate diagnosis, underscoring the significance of CapsNets [29].

4.8 Federated learning

Federated Learning represents a novel paradigm in machine learning that focuses on harnessing vast, decentralized data sprawled across numerous devices or servers to train models [30]. The essence of this approach is its inherent safeguard for privacy; AI models can be developed and fine-tuned without requiring raw data transfer. This becomes indispensable in sectors that handle sensitive information. For instance, in dental caries detection, federated learning stands out as an effective method. This technique can build models using data from dental clinics and hospitals [31]. This is especially remarkable because patient confidentiality remains unassailable even with such extensive data amalgamation, highlighting the immense potential of federated learning in privacy-centric scenarios.

4.9 Multimodal learning

Multimodal Learning is a sophisticated approach in machine learning that thrives on fusing data from diverse modalities, such as text, images, and sound, to refine predictions. This method showcases its strength in dental caries detection by potentially intertwining various strands of information. A typical multimodal learning model can deftly merge dental images with patient medical histories and other pertinent data, paving the way for more precise diagnostic outcomes and better forecasts of disease progression. By harnessing this multifaceted data, practitioners can achieve an enriched understanding, thereby enhancing the overall effectiveness of the diagnostic process [32].

The realm of AI in dental caries detection is poised for transformative progress. While each method has inherent strengths and drawbacks, the selection invariably hinges on the task, the data available, and the unique demands of the challenge. Often, amalgamating various methods can offer the most optimal outcomes. The convergence of burgeoning AI and machine learning innovations with the surge in dental imaging data indicates a trajectory towards highly precise, streamlined, and tailor-made diagnostic techniques. Beyond mere diagnostics, these state-of-the-art tools profoundly elevate the quality of patient care, ushering in a new era for dental health and treatment.

5. Machine learning and image recognition in dental caries

This "data-driven learning" approach has found significant application across the healthcare spectrum, notably in dentistry [33]. Historically, the management of dental caries, particularly its early detection and treatment, has been anchored in clinical evaluations and the interpretation of radiographic images. This method, though adequate to an extent, has its limitations. Subjectivity in interpretations and the potential oversight of nascent caries are notable drawbacks. Enter machine learning and the narrative changes. When exposed to a vast collection of dental images, machine learning algorithms can discern even the subtlest signs of dental caries in their infancy. The efficiency of these models in analyzing and understanding a multitude of images within a short timeframe surpasses human capability, signifying a potential surge in the productivity of dental practices [34].

Supplementing this prowess of machine learning is image recognition. This facet of AI equips machines with a quasi-visual understanding, enabling them to dissect and infer data from images. When it comes to dental caries, this technology becomes invaluable. AI systems harness image recognition to meticulously scan dental radiographs or intraoral photographs, highlighting potential decay sites. The precision of this technology lies in its capability to differentiate between a healthy tooth structure and areas affected by caries, thus streamlining further clinical examinations. Integrating machine learning and image recognition crafts a formidable method for detecting dental caries. The fusion of these technologies ushers in an era of advanced diagnostic instruments characterized by remarkable accuracy and efficiency. It is pivotal to understand that the efficacy of such AI systems is directly proportional to the quality and variety of the training data. A machine learning model exposed to diverse dental images representing various caries stages and a broad patient demographic will likely be the gold standard in reliability.

However, the journey of integrating machine learning and image recognition into dental caries management is full of hurdles. The technological quandary of securing pristine input data and the enigmatic nature of some AI-driven decisions pose challenges. Add to this the ethical conundrums of patient consent and data privacy, and the complexity magnifies. Yet, with adequate safeguards and relentless research, these obstacles are surmountable. The alliance of machine learning and image recognition redefines how dental caries are detected and managed. This transformation promises enhanced diagnostic precision and paves the way for timely and efficacious interventions. As these technologies continue to evolve, it becomes imperative to periodically assess and hone them, ensuring they serve as invaluable adjuncts to the expertise of dental professionals, fostering superior oral healthcare.

5.1 Image processing and analysis techniques for identifying caries lesions

With the rise of digital imaging in dentistry, there has been a growing interest in leveraging image processing and analysis techniques to aid in the early detection and management of dental caries. Early identification of caries lesions can lead to timely intervention, potentially saving the patient from more extensive treatments in the future (**Figure 1**).

5.1.1 Image acquisition

The first step involves acquiring a high-quality image of the tooth or teeth. This could be done using various modalities such as intraoral cameras, digital radiographs, or optical coherence tomography. The quality of the image acquired significantly influences the subsequent analysis; thus, ensuring a clear, high-resolution image is imperative. The process begins with selecting an appropriate imaging modality [35]. Traditional dental radiographs, such as bitewings, periapical, and panoramic images, remain popular due to their comprehensive visualization capabilities. However, intraoral cameras have gained traction for offering a live, high-resolution glimpse into the oral cavity, highlighting potential early-stage caries or enamel anomalies. More recently, Optical Coherence Tomography (OCT) has emerged as a non-invasive technique that captures detailed cross-sectional views of dental structures, thereby aiding in the early identification of caries [36].

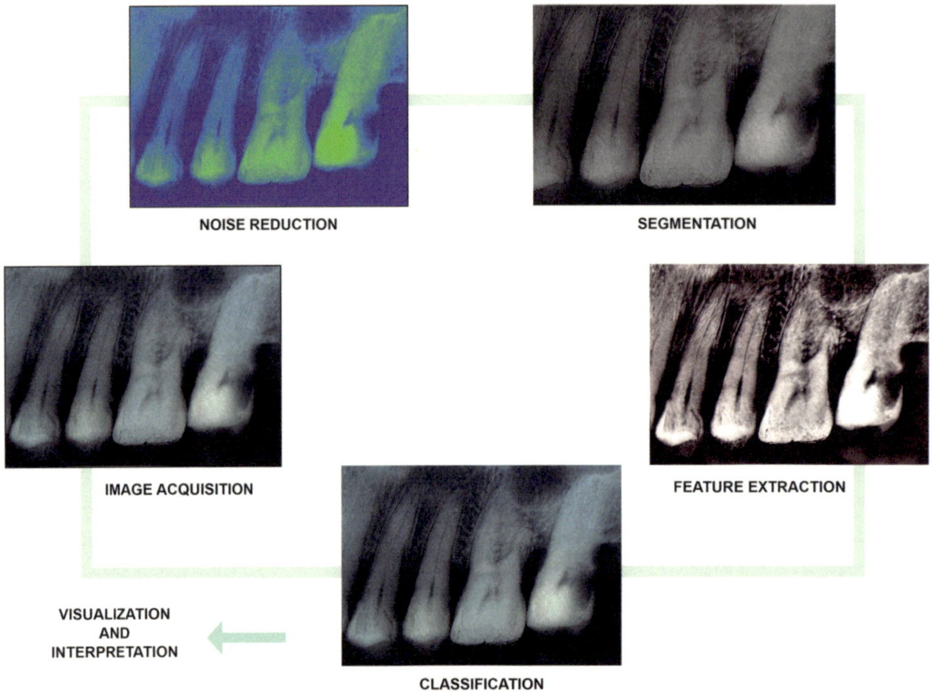

Figure 1.
Dental radiograph analysis and dental caries detection through artificial intelligence.

Quality, especially resolution, is indispensable. While higher resolutions offer detailed insights, revealing even minute structural changes indicative of caries onset, they also pose storage and processing challenges due to larger file sizes. Consistency further accentuates image acquisition, especially when monitoring caries progression or conducting research. Factors like angle, lighting, and imaging settings must remain uniform. Image acquisition in dental caries detection transcends mere picture capturing. It is a meticulous procedure that, when executed with precision, promises an accurate and efficient diagnostic trajectory in the stages that follow.

5.1.2 Pre-processing in dental caries image analysis

The pre-processing stage holds pivotal significance in the dental caries image analysis continuum. It primarily bridges raw image acquisition and intricate analysis, ensuring the input images are refined and optimized for subsequent stages. Dental images, even when captured meticulously, often contain noise, artifacts, or variances in illumination, which can influence the accuracy of caries detection. Pre-processing techniques are designed to mitigate these imperfections and enhance the image's quality [37]. Common methodologies include:

Noise Reduction: Dental images, especially radiographs, can be subjected to random noise due to equipment, transmission errors, or external interferences. Techniques like Gaussian blurring, median filtering, and wavelet denoising are employed to smooth out the image, preserving the essential features while removing extraneous details.

Contrast Enhancement: The image's contrast can be amplified to better visualize dental structures and potential caries lesions. Histogram equalization and adaptive histogram equalization are standard techniques to adjust image contrast, emphasizing subtle differences between healthy and carious dental tissues.

Normalization: Inconsistencies in lighting or image acquisition settings across multiple images can be counteracted by normalizing the intensity levels. This ensures a consistent brightness and contrast range, facilitating comparability across various images.

Segmentation: Only some parts of an image are often relevant for caries detection. Pre-processing may involve segmenting the image, isolating the region of interest (e.g., a specific tooth or quadrant) from the background or adjacent structures. This streamlines the subsequent analysis, focusing only on pertinent areas.

Resolution Scaling: To manage computational efficiency, images may be rescaled to a standardized resolution, especially in AI or machine learning models. This harmonizes the input size for subsequent processing, although care must be taken to ensure that vital diagnostic details are not lost in the rescaling process.

Artifact Removal: Dental images can sometimes contain artifacts - extraneous features or distortions, often arising from equipment malfunctions, patient movement, or external objects (like metal restorations). These artifacts can interfere with accurate caries detection. Pre-processing aims to identify and mitigate these disturbances, ensuring the integrity of the diagnostic image.

The overarching objective of pre-processing is to curate an image that is void of distractions and optimized for clarity. It accentuates the relevant features, equips the image for efficient analysis, and sets the stage for accurate caries detection. As dental imaging evolves with technology's strides, the pre-processing phase will undoubtedly adapt, integrating more sophisticated techniques to ensure that the foundational image quality is preserved and enhanced for crucial diagnostic tasks.

5.1.3 Feature extraction in dental caries image analysis

Feature extraction is a crucial step in the image analysis process, especially in the context of dental caries detection. This phase involves isolating and quantifying pertinent attributes from the pre-processed image, instrumental in characterizing and distinguishing between healthy and carious dental tissues. These attributes or "features" become the foundation upon which classification models make decisions, especially in machine learning or AI-based systems.

5.1.3.1 Texture analysis

Dental caries often manifest changes in the texture of dental tissues. Techniques like gray-level co-occurrence matrix (GLCM), local binary patterns (LBP), and wavelet transforms are employed to extract texture-related features. These methods quantify variations in the image, capturing nuances that can signal the presence of early or advanced carious lesions [38].

5.1.3.2 Shape and morphological features

The contours and morphologies of carious lesions can be distinct from the regular dental anatomy. Edge detection algorithms, such as the Canny or Sobel operators, can help identify the boundaries of lesions. Once the edges are identified, shape descriptors, like compactness, elongation, or roundness, can be calculated to provide insights into the lesion's characteristics.

5.1.3.3 Intensity and statistical features

The pixel intensity distribution within an image or a segmented region can offer valuable information. Mean, variance, skewness, and kurtosis of the pixel intensities can be computed. Carious regions might present with different intensity distributions compared to healthy tissues, making these features valuable for differentiation.

5.1.3.4 Frequency domain features

Transforming the image from the spatial domain to the frequency domain using methods like the Fourier Transform or Wavelet Transform allows the extraction of features that might not be discernible in the standard spatial domain. These frequency-based features can be susceptible to subtle changes caused by caries.

5.1.3.5 Color-based features

While more relevant for intraoral photographs than radiographs, the color attributes of an area can be informative. RGB (Red, Green, Blue) values, Hue-Saturation-Value (HSV) descriptors, or other color spaces can be analyzed to extract features differentiating healthy and carious enamel or dentin.

5.1.3.6 Spatial relationships

In some instances, the relative positioning of features within the dental anatomy can be insightful. For example, the proximity of a potential lesion to known anatomical landmarks, like the enamel-dentin junction, can provide context for the extracted features.

5.1.3.7 Deep learning features

With the advent of deep learning techniques, particularly convolutional neural networks (CNNs), feature extraction can also be automated. In these models, the initial layers often act as feature extractors, identifying and emphasizing attributes of the image that are crucial for caries detection.

Feature extraction transforms an image's rich, intricate details into a structured, quantitative format. These distilled features capture the essence of the image, allowing diagnostic models to efficiently and accurately differentiate between healthy and carious tissues. As image analysis technologies advance, the feature extraction phase will continue to evolve, incorporating more nuanced and sophisticated techniques that elevate the precision and reliability of dental caries detection.

5.1.4 Classification in dental caries image analysis

In dental caries image analysis, classification is the stage where the extracted features from the images are used to categorize or label the data, determining whether a particular region of interest in a dental image is healthy or carious. Given the complexity and variability of oral images, an effective classification system is pivotal for accurate diagnostics [39].

5.1.4.1 Machine learning algorithms

Traditional machine learning techniques have been widely employed for classification tasks in dental imaging. Algorithms such as Support Vector Machines (SVM), Decision Trees, Random Forests, and K-Nearest Neighbors (KNN) can be trained on labeled datasets to recognize patterns in extracted features and classify new, unseen images. Each algorithm offers a distinct approach. For example, SVM works by finding a hyperplane that best separates the classes, while Random Forests employ multiple decision trees to vote on the classification [40].

5.1.4.2 Deep learning and neural networks

In recent years, deep learning, particularly Convolutional Neural Networks (CNNs), has shown promise in dental image classification. CNNs are a subset of neural networks designed to learn spatial hierarchies of features automatically and adaptively from images. They can be trained end-to-end, meaning raw images can be input, and the network handles feature extraction and classification. Due to their depth and complexity, CNNs can capture intricate patterns in images, often outperforming traditional methods, especially when vast amounts of data are available.

5.1.4.3 Ensemble methods

These methods combine multiple classifiers to produce a final decision, typically yielding better performance than individual classifiers. Techniques like bagging, boosting, or stacking can be employed, pooling insights from different models for more robust classification.

5.1.4.4 Evaluation metrics

Once classification models are trained, their performance must be assessed. Metrics such as accuracy, precision, recall, F1-score, and the Area Under the Receiver Operating Characteristic Curve (AUC-ROC) are used. These metrics give insights into the model's actual positive rate, false positive rate, false negatives, and more, facilitating the choice of the most effective classifier for a particular application.

5.1.4.5 Regularization and overfitting

One challenge in classification is overfitting, where the model performs exceptionally well on training data but needs to generalize on unseen data. Techniques such as dropout, L1 or L2 regularization, and early stopping are implemented to ensure robust models generalize well to new data.

5.1.4.6 Transfer learning

Given the challenges in obtaining vast amounts of labeled dental images, transfer learning has emerged as a beneficial approach. Pre-trained models trained on large datasets like ImageNet are fine-tuned on smaller, domain-specific datasets, leveraging the knowledge acquired during the initial training phase to enhance performance in dental caries classification.

5.1.4.7 Continuous learning and model updates

Given the evolving nature of dental imaging and the continuous accrual of new data, classification models should be designed for periodic updates. This ensures they remain current and maintain high-performance levels as new patterns or variations in dental caries emerge.

The classification step in dental caries image analysis is the culmination of all preceding stages. It determines the final diagnostic output, labeling regions as carious or healthy. With the rapid advancements in machine learning and deep learning, classification algorithms are becoming increasingly sophisticated, paving the way for more accurate, efficient, and reliable dental diagnostics.

5.1.4.8 Post-processing

Once the potential caries lesions are identified, post-processing techniques can be used to refine the results. This might involve removing any small, isolated regions identified as caries (which might be false positives) or filling in small gaps in detected caries regions.

5.1.5 Visualization and interpretation

The final processed image is then visualized, highlighting areas detected as caries lesions. Dental professionals can interpret these highlighted areas with clinical knowledge, ensuring the results align with clinical observations and radiographic findings [41]. Image processing and analysis techniques provide a systematic and efficient approach to identifying caries lesions. When combined with the expertise of dental professionals, these techniques can significantly enhance the accuracy of caries detection, leading to better patient outcomes. As technology and algorithms evolve, integrating such techniques in everyday dental practice is set to become more prevalent, revolutionizing the early detection and management of dental caries.

6. Various AI based methods used in the detection of dental caries

6.1 Deep learning for proximal caries detection in bitewings

Proximal dental caries lesions are intricate cavities that develop on the surfaces where teeth come into contact. Their concealed location often makes early detection challenging, leading to a reliance on bitewing radiographs. These radiographs have historically been essential, delivering an in-depth view of the hidden proximal surfaces, including both the maxillary (upper) and mandibular (lower) teeth crown sections. Despite the significant reliance on these radiographs, traditional methods, characterized by visual evaluations and manual image analysis, are susceptible to human subjectivity and potential oversights. The advent of artificial intelligence (AI) and its integration into the healthcare sector heralded a seismic shift in the diagnostic approach to these dental challenges [42]. Deep learning, a sophisticated subset of machine learning, employs multi-layered artificial neural networks to interpret intricate patterns within extensive datasets. These neural networks emulate the complexity and interconnections observed in human neural circuits. In dentistry, deep learning algorithms, especially Convolutional Neural Networks (CNNs), are adept at scrutinizing bitewing radiographs with unmatched precision. The primary aim is to detect proximal caries [43] accurately.

The efficacy of these algorithms is contingent upon rigorous training. An extensive, annotated collection of bitewing images, meticulously marked by seasoned dental experts to indicate caries' presence or absence, serves as the foundational dataset. These models can adeptly analyze new, unlabeled radiographs upon exhaustive training, identifying potential carious patterns based on their learned knowledge [44]. Integrating deep learning offers dual advantages: swift image analysis and mitigating interpretative discrepancies or errors from human fatigue or inherent subjectivity. Contemporary research underscores the unparalleled proficiency of deep learning models, emphasizing their exceptional sensitivity and specificity in detecting proximal caries on bitewing radiographs. In numerous instances, these models rival or surpass the diagnostic acumen of experienced dental professionals [43]. Incorporating deep learning techniques marks a transformative epoch in dental radiographic analysis. By harnessing these avant-garde algorithms, dental practitioners can significantly enhance the precision and efficiency of their diagnoses, culminating in improved patient outcomes and streamlined clinical workflows.

6.2 Deep learning for ICDAS™ classification in bitewing radiographs

The ICDAS™ system, an internationally recognized standard, has ushered in a new era of caries detection and assessment [45]. But with the surge of technological advances, particularly the integration of artificial intelligence, we are on the brink of a revolution in dental diagnostics. Deep learning, characterized by its use of intricate artificial neural networks, can delve deep into extensive datasets, analyzing multiple hidden layers and recognizing nuanced patterns that may elude the human eye. The potency of this technology becomes palpable when applied to bitewing radiographs, the cornerstone of dental imaging. Here, the aim is not just detection but the precise classification of dental caries according to the rigorous benchmarks set by the ICDAS™ system. This level of granularity in diagnostics is pivotal, as it facilitates more personalized treatment plans and proactive interventions.

Central to this endeavor are Convolutional Neural Networks (CNNs). Their architecture makes CNNs uniquely equipped to process visual data, making them the model of choice for imaging-based diagnostics. However, the true efficacy of a CNN is contingent on the quality and comprehensiveness of its training data. An annotated with ICDAS™ scores by expert dental practitioners, a meticulously curated dataset lays the foundation. The rigorous training regimen involves the CNN making predictive inferences on caries classifications, juxtaposed with actual ICDAS™ scores. Discrepancies between predicted and actual scores serve as a feedback mechanism, activating backpropagation algorithms [22]. These algorithms adjust the CNN's parameters, fine-tuning its predictive prowess in a relentless pursuit of diagnostic perfection. Upon satisfactory training, CNN's capabilities are put to the test. Presented with the novel, unlabeled bitewing radiographs, it undertakes the task of discerning and classifying dental caries, assigning them ICDAS™ scores [22]. This marriage of deep learning technology with the ICDAS™ system is emblematic of the future of dental diagnostics — one where precision, consistency, and technology converge to optimize patient outcomes.

6.3 Dental radiographic segmentation with neutrosophic logic

Segmentation of dental radiographic images is pivotal for effective dental caries diagnosis. Traditional methods often grapple with noise and image uncertainties. However, neutrosophic logic presents an innovative solution [46]. Conceived by Florentin Smarandache, this logic comprehends imprecision typical of human cognition and tangible scenarios, surpassing the binary logic's confines of strict truth and falsehood by introducing indeterminacy. When applied to image processing, neutrosophic logic capably navigates radiographic ambiguities. The initial step entails transforming the image to the neutrosophic domain. Pixels are defined by three sets: truth (T), falsehood (F), and indeterminacy (I). These sets reflect the pixel's affiliation to the object (like tooth structure), non-affiliation, and uncertain status [47].

After this transformation, neutrosophic-centric image enhancement methods amplify contrast and minimize noise, heightening structure visibility. Segmentation then employs neutrosophic-designed techniques, utilizing membership degrees within the T, F, and I sets for pixel classification. This neutrosophic segmentation strategy touts several merits, notably its capacity to adeptly manage dental radiographic image uncertainties adeptly, resulting in consistent, precise segmentations, thus refining subsequent analytical procedures [48]. However, it demands significant computational resources, as each pixel requires a three-set analysis. Additionally, selecting optimal parameters for image amplification and segmentation can be intricate, potentially necessitating expert insight. Nevertheless, neutrosophic logic in dental radiographic image segmentation offers a groundbreaking, dependable methodology, propelling advancements in dental ailment detection and diagnostics.

6.4 YOLOv3 and ICCMS™ in bitewing radiographs

YOLO, standing for "You Only Look Once," represents the forefront of object detection in computer vision. Its third version, YOLOv3, offers unmatched speed and accuracy, opening new doors across various detection scenarios. One field ripe for innovation is dentistry, where YOLOv3's capability for accurately detecting and classifying dental caries is now being explored. YOLOv3's adaptation is based on the comprehensive ICCMS™ (International Caries Classification and Management System) radiographic scoring system [49].

YOLOv3, a deep-learning gem, is designed for rapid and sharp object detection. Its efficiency stems from its regressive method, marking objects and predicting class probabilities straight from an image in one step. To align YOLOv3 with dental caries detection, it is trained on a vast bitewing radiographic dataset annotated with caries details and matching ICCMS™ scores. As YOLOv3 trains, it recognizes the visual markers linked to different stages of caries as classified by ICCMS™. In practice, the trained model identifies and matches caries with ICCMS™ scores, annotating a radiograph with accurate caries borders and classifications [50]. YOLOv3's effectiveness in this application is gauged using metrics like precision, recall, F1-score, and mAP, which collectively shed light on its skill in identifying and categorizing dental caries. However, the pathway to embed YOLOv3 in dental diagnostics is challenging. Collecting an extensive, diverse, and well-annotated training dataset is a significant hurdle. YOLOv3's inherent "black box" nature, typical of many deep learning models, can raise questions about its decision-making transparency. This method emphasizes YOLOv3's transformative capability in dental caries detection, particularly its alignment with the ICCMS™ system. While obstacles remain, the convergence of YOLOv3 and ICCMS™ paints a bright picture for the future of dental diagnostics [51].

6.5 Blob detection in dental caries diagnostics

The dawn of blob detection in dental diagnostics represents a paradigm shift in how dental caries are identified and diagnosed. This technique, rooted in image processing, recognizes and distinguishes regions termed 'blobs' based on their unique brightness attributes. In dental radiographs, these blobs are often discerned as shadowy indicators of dental caries, contrasting vividly against the healthier parts of tooth structures [52]. The merits of blob detection in dentistry are multifaceted. Firstly, its precision is noteworthy. The technique's ability to pinpoint even the most nascent lesions facilitates prompt interventions, potentially halting further tooth damage. Then comes the aspect of efficiency. Traditionally, dental professionals might invest significant time in meticulously examining radiographs. With blob detection, this analysis is streamlined, allowing dentists to channel more of their time and focus on direct patient care. Another pivotal advantage is the promise of consistency. By shifting diagnosis to an algorithm-driven approach, the interpretation process sidesteps individual professionals' personal biases and nuances, ensuring a standardized evaluation.

The procedure of blob detection in dental diagnostics unfolds systematically. Initially, radiographs are subjected to pre-processing, where they undergo optimization for contrast and noise reduction. This stage is foundational, priming the images for the rigorous blob identification that follows. The actual process of blob detection sees specialized algorithms deployed to scan the radiograph meticulously. The objective is to highlight areas exhibiting pronounced brightness disparities. As these darker regions come into focus, they are typically flagged as indicators of decay [53]. The concluding phase, post-processing, plays a critical role. Here, the detected blobs are assessed for validity. Determinations are drawn regarding whether they genuinely represent caries, gauging their severity and even predicting potential progression trajectories based on the characteristics of these blobs.

A fascinating frontier in this domain is the burgeoning synergy between blob detection and machine learning. Merging the pinpoint accuracy of blob detection with the dynamic adaptability of machine learning paints a promising picture for dental diagnostics. The combined prowess promises speed and heightened accuracy, and uniformity in diagnosis. And while integrating these technologies is not without its challenges, their combined potential to redefine the landscape of dental care is undeniably vast. As a relatively recent entrant in dental diagnostics, blob detection is rapidly becoming an invaluable tool [54]. With its continued integration with technologies like machine learning, the future of dental diagnostics and care seems poised for significant innovation and patient-centric advancements.

6.6 Dental caries detection with meta-heuristic-based ResNeXt-RNN

The innovative fusion of the ResNeXt-RNN model emerges as a trailblazer in dental caries detection. Building on the foundational prowess of deep learning, the ResNeXt architecture distinguishes itself in managing high-dimensional data sets, especially intricate images. A breakthrough conceptualized by Ramana Kumari, Nagaraja Rao, and Ramana Reddy [55], ResNeXt introduces "cardinality" as an added dimension, augmenting the conventional depth and width dimensions that define neural architectures. But the genius does not stop here. The Recurrent Neural Network (RNN) component is integrated into this image processing. Historically recognized for its aptitude in managing sequences and retaining memory states, RNN offers the ability to analyze temporal dynamics, a particularly crucial facet for assessing the progression of dental conditions over time.

The synergy of ResNeXt and RNN culminates in a model that excels on dual fronts. While the ResNeXt component meticulously captures spatial intricacies, the RNN counterpart evaluates the temporal evolution of dental caries. Elevating this amalgamation further is the integration of meta-heuristic algorithms. These advanced computational blueprints enhance and guide models' learning trajectories, amplifying their overall performance. The methodology unfolds systematically [56]. Dental images are first channeled into the ResNeXt component, which performs the initial feature extraction phase, identifying critical markers that might indicate the presence of caries. These features, once isolated, are directed to the RNN module, which assesses their temporal dynamics – invaluable insights, particularly for studies tracking the longitudinal progression of caries. Simultaneously, the inherent meta-heuristic algorithm plays its part in fine-tuning and optimizing the model's learning parameters.

While the merits of this integrated approach are manifold, promising a panoramic and dynamic view of dental caries detection, it is full of challenges. The complexity inherent in the model might raise interpretability issues. Validating its decisions could become an intricate task. Additionally, sourcing a rich repository of high-quality dental images for training is not only a logistical challenge but also broaches concerns related to patient privacy. Yet, optimism and anticipation are the overarching sentiments surrounding the meta-heuristic-based ResNeXt-RNN model. Its unparalleled capabilities in dental image analysis herald a potential paradigm shift, particularly for early-stage caries detection. As the confluence between AI and dentistry deepens, it is becoming evident that models like these will profoundly shape the future contours of oral health diagnostics.

6.7 PaXNet: Ensemble and capsule classifier for panoramic X-ray caries detection

The application of artificial intelligence (AI) in dentistry has been transformative. One standout model demonstrating its prowess in this domain is PaXNet. This innovative technique leverages Ensemble Transfer Learning and the Capsule Classifier to optimize dental caries detection in panoramic X-rays. PaXNet is a custom-built AI model to identify dental caries using panoramic X-rays [57]. Its two-fold system magnifies the advantages of Ensemble Transfer Learning and Capsule Networks. The former, Ensemble Transfer Learning, amalgamates insights from various pre-trained deep learning models, re-purposing them for dental caries detection. Such integration ensures that the model extracts the most salient features across multiple datasets, augmenting its predictive prowess and adaptability. Conversely, Capsule Networks (CapsNets) introduce a revolutionary neural network structure. They retain nuanced information about the spatial hierarchies and relationships within the features of an image. A Capsule Classifier, built atop the CapsNets, classifies images based on the calculated probabilities of specific feature presence [58].

Within PaXNet, Ensemble Transfer Learning takes the lead, teasing out relevant features from panoramic X-ray captures. Subsequently, these features undergo evaluation by the Capsule Classifier, determining the presence or absence of dental caries. A notable advantage of PaXNet is its capability to identify intricate feature interrelationships within panoramic X-ray images—details that often elude conventional convolutional neural networks. This intrinsic strength translates to enhanced accuracy and precision in caries detection. Empirical evidence supports PaXNet's prowess. Comparative studies have underscored its superior sensitivity, specificity, and accuracy vis-à-vis other machine learning paradigms. Given its formidable performance metrics, PaXNet is preferred for dental healthcare setups. It offers a swift and dependable adjunct opinion on dental caries, streamlining diagnostic processes. PaXNet's synergistic utilization of Ensemble Transfer Learning and Capsule Classifier signifies a watershed moment in dental caries detection from panoramic X-rays [27]. Embracing its potential and mitigating its challenges, we can anticipate PaXNet to redefine dental diagnostic protocols, fostering enhanced patient care trajectories.

6.8 Pervasive deep gradient-based LeNet

The transformative "Pervasive Deep Gradient-Based LeNet Classifier" stands as a beacon in the evolving landscape of dental caries detection, signaling a departure from traditional diagnostic methods. Initially designed by Yann LeCun for character recognition, the LeNet structure, with its specialized convolutional layers, has proven invaluable in processing dental imagery and capturing intricate spatial data hierarchies. Transitioning seamlessly through its layers, from convolutional and pooling stages to a SoftMax classifier, LeNet provides a comprehensive image analysis.

In dental diagnostics, this specific iteration of LeNet has been meticulously tailored. Equipped with an uncanny ability to parse nuanced patterns within data, it scrutinizes dental images precisely, distinguishing pivotal features and subsequently classifying them based on the presence or absence of caries [59]. The model's integration of the "pervasive deep gradient-based" methodology is particularly noteworthy. This technique employs gradient descent, a cornerstone of machine learning optimization, to iteratively refine the model's parameters, ensuring its diagnostic accuracy improves with each training cycle. Among its salient strengths, the model boasts an unparalleled prowess in data management. It can deftly navigate extensive dental image datasets, rendering manual feature extraction a relic of the past. Its operational speed and diagnostic precision allow for swift and accurate disease identification, paving the way for timely and effective treatments. Furthermore, its heightened sensitivity ensures the detection of even the most subtle structural tooth changes, often identifying caries in their initial stages when they are most amenable to treatment. The introduction of the "Pervasive Deep Gradient-Based LeNet Classifier" into the field of dental diagnostics heralds a new era, one in which carries detection becomes increasingly efficient, predictive oral health measures are refined, and overall patient care standards soar to new heights [60].

6.9 AssistDent®: aI-assisted dental diagnostics

AssistDent® is a cutting-edge AI software tailored for precise dental caries detection. Utilizing deep learning algorithms, particularly Convolutional Neural Networks (CNNs), it excels in analyzing dental images, ensuring dental professionals can make informed decisions quickly and accurately. The strength of AssistDent® stems from its ability to scrutinize dental radiographs with unparalleled precision. These capabilities arise from extensive training on numerous dental radiographs annotated by seasoned professionals. As a result, the early stages of dental caries are quickly identified, making early intervention feasible. The software's intuitive interface seamlessly integrates into a dental clinic's workflow, offering real-time feedback that revolutionizes the diagnostic process, giving practitioners more time with their patients. Rigorous tests confirm AssistDent®'s exemplary sensitivity and specificity in caries detection, further establishing its role as an indispensable tool for dental diagnostics [61, 62].

However, like most AI tools, AssistDent® has its challenges. Its efficacy is largely contingent upon the quality of its training data, emphasizing the need for ongoing updates and training with diverse datasets. Efforts to enhance its transparency and interpretability in decision-making are continuous. Looking to the future, the potential for AssistDent® extends beyond merely caries detection. As AI evolves and datasets grow, it is poised to become a holistic diagnostic powerhouse for a spectrum of oral conditions. In essence, AssistDent® embodies the next giant leap in AI-enhanced dental care, pointing towards a future where diagnostics are more refined, swift, and universally accessible.

6.10 Bitewing radiographs: deep learning caries classification with ICDAS™

Deep learning algorithms have seen a rising application in identifying and classifying dental caries in bitewing radiographs, mainly using the globally acknowledged ICDAS™ (International Caries Detection and Assessment System) radiographic scoring. This system standardizes caries detection, allowing more streamlined communication among dental professionals. Within the ICDAS™ framework, dental caries is scored on a spectrum from 0 to 6, with 0 denoting sound tooth surfaces and six pointing to pronounced cavities [63]. Deep learning, an advanced branch of machine learning, employs artificial neural networks with numerous hidden layers, enabling intricate pattern recognition from vast datasets. Within dental diagnostics, this technology can be tailored to sift through bitewing radiographs and categorize dental caries based on the ICDAS™ criteria. Convolutional neural networks (CNNs), a type of deep learning model, play a pivotal role due to their aptitude for visual data analysis, making them ideal for image-centric tasks.

The initial step to developing such a model demands a comprehensive dataset of annotated bitewing radiographs. Expert dental professionals must meticulously label each radiograph with its corresponding ICDAS™ score. During the training phase, the CNN evolves, recognizing radiographic patterns that align with each specific ICDAS™ grade [64]. This learning is facilitated by a mechanism known as backpropagation. Here, the model's predictions are juxtaposed against actual labels, and subsequent adjustments are made to minimize discrepancies. After this rigorous training, the model can autonomously assign ICDAS™ scores to previously unanalyzed bitewing radiographs.

7. Ethical and clinical considerations

A significant cornerstone of any AI system is the vast troves of data it feeds on. This encompasses a wide range of patient-specific data in dentistry: from dental records and radiographic images to detailed medical histories. Acquiring this data mandates an informed consent process, where patients are fully aware of their data's utilization, storage, and potential risks. The subsequent storage of such critical information raises concerns about encryption, unauthorized access, and potential breaches. In today's interconnected digital era, data often traverses various platforms, sometimes extending to third-party vendors. This sharing must stringently align with privacy regulations like GDPR or HIPAA, ensuring uncompromised patient confidentiality. Moreover, anonymizing data for AI model training can further mitigate identification risks.

The potential of AI in revolutionizing dental care pivots on its accuracy and reliability. The backbone of an accurate AI system is the quality of its training data, which must be comprehensive, varied, and genuinely representative of diverse patient demographics to prevent inherent biases and inaccuracies. Rigorous validation processes, where AI outcomes are juxtaposed against traditional diagnostic results, are imperative to vouch for the system's consistency. A challenge often surfaces with AI is its opaque "black box" algorithms, which can hinder a field where traceability and understandability of diagnoses are crucial [65]. Thus, fostering transparency and promoting an environment where AI acts as an assistant to human expertise rather than a replacement can be instrumental. The horizon of AI in dental caries management is undeniably promising. However, its seamless and efficacious integration into the dental sphere demands meticulous navigation of the intertwined ethical and clinical pathways. Addressing these considerations will maximize AI's potential and elevate the dental care standard, blending technology and human expertise in a harmonious symphony.

8. Limitations and challenges

The infiltration of Artificial Intelligence (AI) into the intricate dental caries diagnosis and management domain promises a transformative impact. But like any innovation, AI faces its set of hurdles. These challenges, ranging from technical to human, underscore the need for careful deployment of AI tools while maintaining a balanced perspective on their role in dental care. One predominant challenge is the variability in AI-driven results. AI models, especially when delving into nuanced realms like dental caries detection, may sometimes produce inconsistent or variable outcomes, depending on the algorithm's design or the data it was trained on. These inconsistencies could lead to missed diagnoses or false positives, which can have considerable ramifications in the sensitive patient care environment. Clinicians might find themselves at crossroads, especially when the AI output deviates from their clinical judgment, potentially leading to decision-making dilemmas [16].

At the heart of any effective AI system lies its data – the more robust and diverse, the better. However, AI's dependence on the quality and quantity of data presents a significant challenge. Incomplete, biased, or unrepresentative datasets can skew AI outputs, rendering them less accurate or misleading. In dental caries, where variances can be subtle, training AI models on limited or non-diverse data can gravely compromise their detection capabilities [66]. The quest for substantial, high-quality data is thus not just a technical requisite but a critical determinant of the AI system's clinical utility. But perhaps one of the most profound challenges springs not from technology but from its human stakeholders. The dental community, built on years of rigorous training and honed expertise, might view AI's advent with skepticism or even resistance. The essence of dental care goes beyond mere diagnoses – it encompasses the human touch, experience-based intuition, and a relationship of trust with patients. To many in the dental fraternity, relegating some of these responsibilities to an algorithm might seem disconcerting. Striking a harmonious balance between human expertise and automation is essential. AI should be perceived not as a replacement but as a tool – an adjunct that augments the dentist's capabilities, making their practice more efficient and precise. The promise held by AI in reshaping dental caries management is immense, but it is crucial to approach this frontier with cognizance of its limitations [67]. The true potential of AI in dental care can be realized by addressing these challenges head-on and fostering a collaborative spirit between technology and human expertise.

9. The future of AI in dental caries management

The relentless march of technological progress, coupled with the ever-evolving field of artificial intelligence (AI), heralds an exciting new era for dental care. As AI continues to weave its way into myriad aspects of healthcare, dental caries management stands to benefit enormously. The current landscape of dental caries management has already seen revolutionary changes with the integration of AI, especially in detection. The future, however, is even more promising. Advanced AI algorithms are projected to achieve unparalleled accuracy in spotting early signs of dental caries, reducing the chances of false negatives, and ensuring timely interventions. As AI systems continue to 'learn' from an expanding database of dental images and case studies, their predictive capabilities will be refined further. This implies that, in the future, AI might not just identify existing caries but also predict potential decay based on a combination of the patient's oral history, habits, and genetic predispositions [68].

Moreover, management tools are expected to evolve, integrating real-time feedback mechanisms. Imagine a scenario where, during a dental procedure, an AI-powered tool offers real-time guidance to a dentist, suggesting optimal interventions based on the analysis of thousands of similar cases. Such advancements can drastically reduce procedural errors and improve treatment outcomes. AI's potential is not restricted to stand-alone applications. Its true power might be unleashed when integrated with other emerging dental technologies. Integrating AI with tele-dentistry platforms can democratize dental care, especially in remote regions. AI-powered diagnostic tools can offer preliminary assessments, guiding patients in areas without immediate dental expertise and suggesting when to seek advanced care. The future seems bright as AI matures and finds its footing in dental care. From advanced detection tools to create a comprehensive, patient-centric care model, AI promises to reshape the fabric of dental caries management, steering it towards excellence and holistic well-being.

Conflict of interest

The authors declare no conflict of interest.

Author details

Sukumaran Anil[1*], Krishnaa Sudeep[2], Sudeep Saratchandran[2]
and Vishnupriya K. Sweety[3]

1 Department of Dentistry, Oral Health Institute, Hamad Medical Corporation, Doha, Qatar

2 PMS College of Dental Science and Research, Trivandrum, Kerala, India

3 Pushpagiri Institute of Medical Sciences and Research Centre, Kerala, India

*Address all correspondence to: drsanil@gmail.com

References

[1] Watt RG, Daly B, Allison P, Macpherson LMD, Venturelli R, Listl S, et al. Ending the neglect of global oral health: Time for radical action. Lancet. 2019;**394**:261-272. DOI: 10.1016/S0140-6736(19)31133-X

[2] Chen X, Daliri EB, Kim N, Kim JR, Yoo D, Oh DH. Microbial Etiology and prevention of dental caries: Exploiting natural products to inhibit cariogenic biofilms. Pathogens. 2020;**9**:569. Epub 20200714. DOI: 10.3390/pathogens9070569

[3] Silverstone LM, Hicks MJ, Featherstone MJ. Dynamic factors affecting lesion initiation and progression in human dental enamel. II. Surface morphology of sound enamel and carieslike lesions of enamel. Quintessence International. 1988;**19**:773-785

[4] Ding H, Wu J, Zhao W, Matinlinna JP, Burrow MF, Tsoi JKH. Artificial intelligence in dentistry—A review. Frontiers in Dental Medicine. 2023;**4**:1-13. DOI: 10.3389/fdmed.2023.1085251

[5] Nguyen TT, Larrivee N, Lee A, Bilaniuk O, Durand R. Use of artificial intelligence in dentistry: Current clinical trends and research advances. Journal of the Canadian Dental Association. 2021;**87**:l7

[6] Kelly CJ, Karthikesalingam A, Suleyman M, Corrado G, King D. Key challenges for delivering clinical impact with artificial intelligence. BMC Medicine. 2019;**17**:195. Epub 20191029. DOI: 10.1186/s12916-019-1426-2

[7] Selwitz RH, Ismail AI, Pitts NB. Dental caries. Lancet. 2007;**369**:51-59. DOI: 10.1016/S0140-6736(07)60031-2

[8] Macey R, Walsh T, Riley P, Glenny AM, Worthington HV, O'Malley L, et al. Visual or visual-tactile examination to detect and inform the diagnosis of enamel caries. Cochrane Database of Systematic Reviews. 2021;**6**:CD014546. Epub 20210614. DOI: 10.1002/14651858.CD014546

[9] Ding B, Zhang Z, Liang Y, Wang W, Hao S, Meng Z, et al. Detection of dental caries in oral photographs taken by mobile phones based on the YOLOv3 algorithm. Annals of Translational Medicine. 2021;**9**:1622. DOI: 10.21037/atm-21-4805

[10] Grieco P, Jivraj A, Da Silva J, Kuwajima Y, Ishida Y, Ogawa K, et al. Importance of bitewing radiographs for the early detection of interproximal carious lesions and the impact on healthcare expenditure in Japan. Annals of Translational Medicine. 2022;**10**:2. DOI: 10.21037/atm-21-2197

[11] Oh SH, Lee SR, Choi JY, Choi YS, Kim SH, Yoon HC, et al. Detection of dental caries and cracks with quantitative light-induced fluorescence in comparison to radiographic and visual examination: A retrospective case study. Sensors (Basel). 2021;**21**:1741. Epub 20210303. DOI: 10.3390/s21051741

[12] Serban C, Lungeanu D, Bota SD, Cotca CC, Negrutiu ML, Duma VF, et al. Emerging technologies for dentin caries detection—a systematic review and meta-analysis. Journal of Clinical Medicine. 2022;**11**:1-23. Epub 20220128. DOI: 10.3390/jcm11030674

[13] Chong MJ, Seow WK, Purdie DM, Cheng E, Wan V. Visual-tactile examination compared with conventional radiography, digital

radiography, and Diagnodent in the diagnosis of occlusal occult caries in extracted premolars. Pediatric Dentistry. 2003;**25**:341-349

[14] Carrillo-Perez F, Pecho OE, Morales JC, Paravina RD, Della Bona A, Ghinea R, et al. Applications of artificial intelligence in dentistry: A comprehensive review. Journal of Esthetic and Restorative Dentistry. 2022;**34**:259-280. Epub 20211129. DOI: 10.1111/jerd.12844

[15] Vishwanathaiah S, Fageeh HN, Khanagar SB, Maganur PC. Artificial intelligence its uses and application in Pediatric dentistry: A review. Biomedicine. 2023;**11**:788. Epub 20230305. DOI: 10.3390/biomedicines11030788

[16] Patil S, Albogami S, Hosmani J, Mujoo S, Kamil MA, Mansour MA, et al. Artificial intelligence in the diagnosis of oral diseases: Applications and pitfalls. Diagnostics (Basel). 2022;**12**:1-14. Epub 20220419. DOI: 10.3390/diagnostics12051029

[17] Mahdi SS, Battineni G, Khawaja M, Allana R, Siddiqui MK, Agha D. How does artificial intelligence impact digital healthcare initiatives? A review of AI applications in dental healthcare. International Journal of Information Management Data Insights. 2023;**3**:100144. DOI: 10.1016/j.jjimei.2022.100144

[18] Bohr A, Memarzadeh K, editors. The rise of artificial intelligence in healthcare applications. Artificial Intelligence in Healthcare. Academic Press; 2020. pp. 25-60. ISBN 9780128184387. DOI: 10.1016/B978-0-12-818438-7.00002-2

[19] Ren R, Luo H, Su C, Yao Y, Liao W. Machine learning in dental, oral and craniofacial imaging: A review of recent progress. PeerJ. 2021;**9**:e11451. Epub 20210517. DOI: 10.7717/peerj.11451

[20] Kokomoto K, Okawa R, Nakano K, Nozaki K. Intraoral image generation by progressive growing of generative adversarial network and evaluation of generated image quality by dentists. Scientific Reports. 2021;**11**:18517. Epub 20210916. DOI: 10.1038/s41598-021-98043-3

[21] Farhadian M, Shokouhi P, Torkzaban P. A decision support system based on support vector machine for diagnosis of periodontal disease. BMC Research Notes. 2020;**13**:337. Epub 20200713. DOI: 10.1186/s13104-020-05180-5

[22] Yamashita R, Nishio M, Do RKG, Togashi K. Convolutional neural networks: An overview and application in radiology. Insights Into Imaging. 2018;**9**:611-629. Epub 20180622. DOI: 10.1007/s13244-018-0639-9

[23] Yang Y-H, Kim J-S, Jeong S-H. Prediction of dental caries in 12-year-old children using machine-learning algorithms. Journal of Korean Academy of Oral Health. 2020;**44**:55-63. DOI: 10.11149/jkaoh.2020.44.1.55

[24] Breiman L. Random forests. Machine Learning. 2001;**45**:5-32. DOI: 10.1023/a:1010933404324

[25] Oztekin F, Katar O, Sadak F, Aydogan M, Yildirim TT, Plawiak P, et al. Automatic semantic segmentation for dental restorations in panoramic radiography images using U-net model. International Journal of Imaging Systems and Technology. 2022;**32**:1990-2001. DOI: 10.1002/ima.22803

[26] Taleb A, Rohrer C, Bergner B, De Leon G, Rodrigues JA, Schwendicke F, et al. Self-supervised learning methods

for label-efficient dental caries classification. Diagnostics (Basel). 2022;**12**:1-15. Epub 20220516. DOI: 10.3390/diagnostics12051237

[27] Qayyum A, Tahir A, Butt MA, Luke A, Abbas HT, Qadir J, et al. Dental caries detection using a semi-supervised learning approach. Scientific Reports. 2023;**13**:749. Epub 20230113. DOI: 10.1038/s41598-023-27808-9

[28] Tang B, Li A, Li B, Wang M. CapSurv: Capsule network for survival analysis with whole slide pathological images. IEEE Access. 2019;**7**:26022-26030. DOI: 10.1109/access.2019.2901049

[29] Sabour S, Frosst N, Hinton GE. Dynamic routing between capsules. In: Proceedings of the 31st International Conference on Neural Information Processing Systems. Long Beach, California, USA: Curran Associates Inc.; 2017. pp. 3859-3869

[30] Rischke R, Schneider L, Muller K, Samek W, Schwendicke F, Krois J. Federated learning in dentistry: Chances and challenges. Journal of Dental Research. 2022;**101**:1269-1273. Epub 20220731. DOI: 10.1177/00220345221108953

[31] Schwendicke F, Cejudo Grano de Oro J, Garcia Cantu A, Meyer-Lueckel H, Chaurasia A, Krois J. Artificial intelligence for caries detection: Value of data and information. Journal of Dental Research. 2022;**101**:1350-1356. Epub 20220822. DOI: 10.1177/00220345221113756

[32] Zhao D, Homayounfar M, Zhen Z, Wu MZ, Yu SY, Yiu KH, et al. A multimodal deep learning approach to predicting systemic diseases from Oral conditions. Diagnostics (Basel). 2022;**12**:3192. Epub 20221216. DOI: 10.3390/diagnostics12123192

[33] Kang I-A, Ngnamsie Njimbouom S, Lee K-O, Kim J-D. DCP: Prediction of dental caries using machine learning in personalized medicine. Applied Sciences. 2022;**12**:3043. DOI: 10.3390/app12063043

[34] AbuSalim S, Zakaria N, Islam MR, Kumar G, Mokhtar N, Abdulkadir SJ. Analysis of deep learning techniques for dental informatics: A systematic literature review. Healthcare (Basel). 2022;**10**:1892. Epub 20220928. DOI: 10.3390/healthcare10101892

[35] Kuhnisch J, Meyer O, Hesenius M, Hickel R, Gruhn V. Caries detection on intraoral images using artificial intelligence. Journal of Dental Research. 2022;**101**:158-165. Epub 20210820. DOI: 10.1177/00220345211032524

[36] Shimada Y, Sadr A, Sumi Y, Tagami J. Application of optical coherence tomography (OCT) for diagnosis of caries, cracks, and defects of restorations. Current Oral Health Reports. 2015;**2**:73-80. DOI: 10.1007/s40496-015-0045-z

[37] Sukanya A, Krishnamurthy K, Balakrishnan T. Comparison of pre-processing techniques for dental image analysis. Current Medical Imaging. 2020;**16**:776-780. DOI: 10.2174/1573405615666191115101536

[38] Geetha V, Aprameya K. Textural analysis based classification of digital X-ray images for dental caries diagnosis. International Journal of Engineering Manufacturing (IJEM). 2019;**9**:44-45

[39] Sonavane A, Yadav R, Khamparia A. Dental cavity classification of using convolutional neural network. IOP Conference Series: Materials Science and Engineering. 2021;**1022**:012116. DOI: 10.1088/1757-899x/1022/1/012116

[40] Ambika P. In: Raj P, Evangeline P, editors. The Digital Twin Paradigm for

Smarter Systems and Environments: The Industry Use Cases. Amsterdam, Netherlands: Elsevier; 2020. pp. 321-338. DOI: 10.1016/bs.adcom.2019.10.007

[41] Mertens S, Krois J, Cantu AG, Arsiwala LT, Schwendicke F. Artificial intelligence for caries detection: Randomized trial. Journal of Dentistry. 2021;**115**:103849. Epub 20211014. DOI: 10.1016/j.jdent.2021.103849

[42] Shah N, Bansal N, Logani A. Recent advances in imaging technologies in dentistry. World Journal of Radiology. 2014;**6**:794-807. DOI: 10.4329/wjr.v6.i10.794

[43] Chen X, Guo J, Ye J, Zhang M, Liang Y. Detection of proximal caries lesions on bitewing radiographs using deep learning method. Caries Research. 2022;**56**:455-463. Epub 20221010. DOI: 10.1159/000527418

[44] Lee S, Oh SI, Jo J, Kang S, Shin Y, Park JW. Deep learning for early dental caries detection in bitewing radiographs. Scientific Reports. 2021;**11**:16807. Epub 20210819. DOI: 10.1038/s41598-021-96368-7

[45] Gugnani N, Pandit IK, Srivastava N, Gupta M, Sharma M. International caries detection and assessment system (ICDAS): A new concept. International Journal of Clinical Pediatric Dentistry. 2011;**4**:93-100. Epub 20100415. DOI: 10.5005/jp-journals-10005-1089

[46] Datta S, Chaki N, Modak B. A novel technique for dental radiographic image segmentation based on neutrosophic logic. Decision Analytics Journal. 2023;**7**:100223. DOI: 10.1016/j.dajour.2023.100223

[47] Nagarajan D, Broum S. Neutrosophic DICOM image processing and its applications. Neutrosophic Sets and Systems. 2023;**53**:21

[48] Luo D, Zeng W, Chen J, Tang W. Deep learning for automatic image segmentation in stomatology and its clinical application. Frontiers in Medical Technology. 2021;**3**:767836. Epub 20211213. DOI: 10.3389/fmedt.2021.767836

[49] Panyarak W, Suttapak W, Wantanajittikul K, Charuakkra A, Prapayasatok S. Assessment of YOLOv3 for caries detection in bitewing radiographs based on the ICCMS radiographic scoring system. Clinical Oral Investigations. 2023;**27**:1731-1742. Epub 20221128. DOI: 10.1007/s00784-022-04801-6

[50] Juyal A, Tiwari H, Singh UK, Kumar N, Kumar S. Dental caries detection using faster R-CNN and YOLO V3. In: ITM Web of Conferences. Les Ulis, France: EDP Sciences; 2023. p. 02005

[51] Salahin SMS, Ullaa MDS, Ahmed S, Mohammed N, Farook TH, Dudley J. One-stage methods of computer vision object detection to classify carious lesions from smartphone imaging. Oral. 2023;**3**:176-190. DOI: 10.3390/oral3020016

[52] Majanga V, Viriri S. Automatic blob detection for dental caries. Applied Sciences. 2021;**11**:9232. DOI: 10.3390/app11199232

[53] Osterloh D, Viriri S. Caries detection in non-standardized periapical dental X-rays. In: Computer Aided Intervention and Diagnostics in Clinical and Medical Images. New York, USA: Springer; 2019. pp. 143-152

[54] Xu Y, Wu T, Charlton JR, Gao F, Bennett KM. Small blob detector using Bi-threshold constrained adaptive scales. IEEE Transactions on Biomedical Engineering. 2021;**68**:2654-2665.

Epub 20210823. DOI: 10.1109/TBME.2020.3046252

[55] Kumari AR, Rao SN, Reddy PR. Design of hybrid dental caries segmentation and caries detection with meta-heuristic-based ResneXt-RNN. Biomedical Signal Processing and Control. 2022;**78**:103961

[56] Reddi SK, Babu CR. Meta-heuristic-based hybrid Resnet with recurrent neural network for enhanced stock market prediction. International Journal of Distributed Systems and Technologies (IJDST). 2022;**13**:1-28

[57] Haghanifar A, Majdabadi MM, Haghanifar S, Choi Y, Ko S-B. PaXNet: Tooth segmentation and dental caries detection in panoramic X-ray using ensemble transfer learning and capsule classifier. Multimedia Tools and Applications. 2023;**82**:27659-27679. DOI: 10.1007/s11042-023-14435-9

[58] Mazzia V, Salvetti F, Chiaberge M. Efficient-CapsNet: Capsule network with self-attention routing. Scientific Reports. 2021;**11**:14634. Epub 20210719. DOI: 10.1038/s41598-021-93977-0

[59] Vimalarani G, Ramachandraiah U. Automatic diagnosis and detection of dental caries in bitewing radiographs using pervasive deep gradient based LeNet classifier model. Microprocessors and Microsystems. 2022;**94**:104654

[60] Sivari E, Senirkentli GB, Bostanci E, Guzel MS, Acici K, Asuroglu T. Deep learning in diagnosis of dental anomalies and diseases: A systematic review. Diagnostics (Basel). 2023;**13**:2512. Epub 20230727. DOI: 10.3390/diagnostics13152512

[61] Devlin H, Williams T, Graham J, Ashley M. The ADEPT study: A comparative study of dentists' ability to detect enamel-only proximal caries in bitewing radiographs with and without the use of AssistDent artificial intelligence software. British Dental Journal. 2021;**231**:481-485. Epub 20211022. DOI: 10.1038/s41415-021-3526-6

[62] Anil S, Porwal P, Porwal A. Transforming dental caries diagnosis through artificial intelligence-based techniques. Cureus. 2023;**15**:1-7, e41694. DOI: 10.7759/cureus.41694

[63] Thanh MTG, Van Toan N, Ngoc VTN, Tra NT, Giap CN, Nguyen DM. Deep learning application in dental caries detection using intraoral photos taken by smartphones. Applied Sciences. 2022;**12**:5504. DOI: 10.3390/app12115504

[64] Alzubaidi L, Zhang J, Humaidi AJ, Al-Dujaili A, Duan Y, Al-Shamma O, et al. Review of deep learning: Concepts, CNN architectures, challenges, applications, future directions. Journal of Big Data. 2021;**8**:53. Epub 20210331. DOI: 10.1186/s40537-021-00444-8

[65] Myllyaho L, Raatikainen M, Männistö T, Mikkonen T, Nurminen JK. Systematic literature review of validation methods for AI systems. Journal of Systems and Software. 2021;**181**:111050. DOI: 10.1016/j.jss.2021.111050

[66] Vodanovic M, Subasic M, Milosevic D, Savic PI. Artificial intelligence in medicine and dentistry. Acta Stomatologica Croatica. 2023;**57**:70-84. DOI: 10.15644/asc57/1/8

[67] Agrawal P, Nikhade P. Artificial intelligence in dentistry: Past, present, and future. Cureus. 2022;**14**:e27405. Epub 20220728. DOI: 10.7759/cureus.27405

[68] Pang L, Wang K, Tao Y, Zhi Q, Zhang J, Lin H. A new model for caries risk prediction in teenagers using a machine learning algorithm based on environmental and genetic factors. Frontiers in Genetics. 2021;**12**:636867. Epub 20210311. DOI: 10.3389/fgene.2021.636867

Chapter 4

The Use of Fluoride for Enamel Caries Management in Infants

Ana Cláudia Rodrigues Chibinski, Anna Bárbara Maluf, Larissa Yumi Ito, Letícia Maira Wambier, Mayara Vitorino Gevert and Vitória Monteiro

Abstract

The presence of one or more decayed surfaces (cavitated or non-cavitated), lost or restored (due to caries) in any primary tooth in a child under 6 years old is considered Early Childhood Caries (ECC). Therefore, as soon as an initial enamel caries lesion is detected in a primary tooth, adequate measures must be adopted to halt the progression of this lesion into a cavity. To achieve this objective, fluoridated products are the most common resource, being available worldwide. Considering the age group, the use of fluoridated toothpaste and fluoride varnishes are indicated as simple and effective preventive and therapeutic methods. This chapter will discuss the advantages of these methods based on contemporary scientific evidence, as well as their expected clinical results when properly indicated and used.

Keywords: fluorides, toothpastes, fluoride varnishes, infants, dental caries

1. Introduction

It is expected that more than 530 million children around the world have untreated caries lesions, with the largest number of these lesions concentrated at the age of 5 years old [1]. These lesions are the clinical sign of Early Childhood Caries (ECC), defined as "the presence of one or more decayed surfaces (cavitated or non-cavitated), lost or restored (due to caries) in any primary tooth in a child under 6 years old" [2]. Specifically, in America, data from a systematic review showed a 48% prevalence (CI 95% 42–54) of ECC [3].

Therefore, any clinical evidence of disease activity in babies may be classified as ECC, since a white spot can evolve to cavitation. So, different strategies must be adopted, which include effective procedures for controlling lesions in their different stages of development. Ideally, this disease management should occur before cavitation, preventing the need for restorative treatment and maintaining the integrity of the dental structure.

Considering current knowledge about cariology, the treatment can be done through non-invasive procedures and carious lesions can be controlled before cavitation (primary prevention) [2]. These procedures offer the patient a "friendly" treatment for the child and tooth that prevents further loss of tooth structure, associating home care performed by parents/caregivers with in-office professional care. The aim is to adapt hygiene and diet to control the dysbiosis responsible for dental demineralization, associated with non-invasive methods to remineralize active lesions.

The prevention and treatment of caries disease involve the use of fluoride, which is a substance that interferes in demineralization-remineralization dynamics (DES-RE process). Therefore, fluoride is considered "a therapeutic agent that acts by controlling the beginning and development of caries lesions from the pre-cavitated stage of lesions formation" [4]. After topic application, the fluoride may be present in 5 different sites in the mouth: (1) biofilm and saliva; (2) incorporated into hydroxyapatite crystals into fluorapatite-like crystals; (3) enamel fluid; (4) adsorbed into hydroxyapatite surface, and (5) in the form of calcium fluoride (CaF2) [5]. Furthermore, its action is based on the constant presence of fluoride in the mouth, acting to reduce the demineralization and favoring the remineralization of the tooth. Therefore, the benefit is achieved by local and not systemic action [5], which is why oral fluoride supplementation is not recommended.

The fluor may be administered collectively to the population (fluoridation of public water supply, fluoridated salt, fluoridated milk), individually for self-application (fluoridated toothpaste, fluoridated solutions for mouthwashes), and exclusively for professional use (gels, foams, varnishes, slow-release devices, and fluoride-releasing restorative materials).

The use of fluoride agents in children and adolescents was analyzed by different systematic reviews, and it was concluded that toothpastes [6], fluoride mouthwashes [7], fluoride gel applications [8] and fluoride varnishes [9] are effective in reducing the incidence of caries.

Notwithstanding, not all forms of fluoride administration may be used in babies, safely, for prevention and caries treatment. Despite the patient's risk, fluoridated water and fluoridated toothpaste should be a constant in the baby's daily life. However, additional methods should only be indicated by a professional if an imbalanced condition is present in the baby's oral cavity. Fluoride gels, foams, and mouthwashes are not indicated for use in babies due to the possibility of inadvertent ingestion of the product.

Therefore, in this chapter, the discussion is focused on fluoride toothpaste, the main individual method, and fluoride varnishes, the main professional method, for the use of fluoride in infants.

2. Fluoride toothpaste

The understanding that caries is a biofilm-dependent disease can justify that toothbrushing is an essential process to control dental caries, using the association of systematic disorganization of the biofilm (toothbrushing) with daily topical application of the fluoride present in the toothpaste.

Strong evidence supports the use of fluoride toothpaste for caries prevention [10] with a minimum concentration of 1.000 ppm of Fluor [6]. This protocol was recommended in the Bangkok Declaration to reduce the prevalence of ECC [2].

In addition to the fluoride concentration in the toothpaste, other factors can also influence the use of toothbrushing in the prevention of caries. The best results are obtained with at least two brushings a day [2], and the toothbrushing before bedtime is the most important one because there is a reduction in salivary flow during sleep. It is also advisable not to rinse with water after brushing, as it may reduce the amount of fluoride in the oral cavity.

2.1 Fluoride toothpastes and acute toxicity

The probably toxic fluoride dose is 5.0 mg F/kg of body weight. Therefore, a 2-year-old child weighing approximately 12 kg would only be at risk of acute toxicity if he/she ingests 60 g of fluoride toothpaste with a concentration of 1.000 ppm F, which is more than the whole amount in a tube of toothpaste commonly sold (50 mg) [11]. So, although it is a possibility, it is a quite remote one. Conversely, chronic toxicity (fluorosis) occurs more frequently and it is what will be discussed below.

2.2 Fluoride toothpastes and fluorosis

Children under 5 years old have not yet developed the expectoration reflex and they swallow most of the fluoride in the toothpaste used during toothbrushing. For this reason, for a long time, fluoridated toothpaste and fluoridated water were considered responsible for the prevalence of fluorosis, and the recommendation was to use fluoride-free toothpaste for babies [12].

Currently, the importance of fluoride toothpaste in daily oral hygiene procedures is known, but the dose used in each brushing must be controlled (**Table 1**), since the amount of toothpaste swallowed is inversely proportional to the child's age and directly proportional to the distribution of toothpaste in the toothbrush [14].

The use of fluoridated dentifrices in babies is based on the concept that the benefit in controlling dental caries is obtained with a minimum risk for the development of fluorosis. There is a "window of susceptibility" for the occurrence of dental fluorosis,

Age	Weight	Erupted Teeth	Amount of toothpaste per brushing	Amount of soluble fluoride per brushing	Daily dose to 2 brushes	% limited dose*
1 year	10 kg	4–8 incisive	0,05 g like a half-rice grain 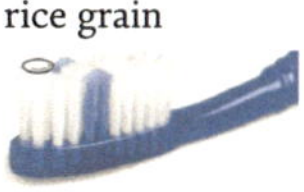	0,055 g	0,011 mg F/kg/day	16%
2 years	12,5 kg	All the incisives	0,1 g like a rice grain 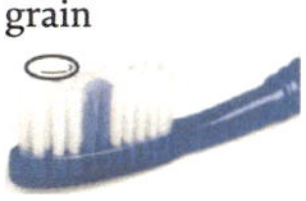	0,11 g	0,0176 mg F/kg/day	25%
5–6 years	20 kg	All primaries teeth	0,3 g like a pea grain 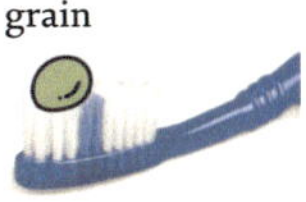	0,33 g	0,033 mg F/kg/day	47%

* *Adapted from [13].*

Table 1.
Use of fluoride dentifrices with 1.100 ppm in the first years of life and the risk of dental fluorosis.

which is the period that coincides with enamel formation. For most permanent teeth, this occurs in the first 6 to 8 years of a child's life, with the exception of permanent incisors, when it corresponds to the first 3 years of a baby's life [15]. Therefore, since the birth of the first deciduous tooth, when brushing with fluoridated dentifrices is implemented, until approximately 8 years old, constant supervision is important to minimize swallowing while maintaining effective exposure to fluoride. Using the correct amount of toothpaste on the toothbrush, even if it is ingested (which is common in babies), the daily limit of systemic fluoride needed to develop fluorosis is not reached (**Table 1**).

Association with additional sources of fluoride like fluoridated water, may result in levels capable of causing fluorosis. However, it has been observed in most of the studied populations that if fluorosis develops, it is very mild, with little importance for the esthetics and quality of life of patients [16].

An important advice during this step is to guide parents/caregivers about the correct amount of toothpaste in each brushing according to the baby's age group. Often, the description used by the dentist may not be correctly interpreted by parents/caregivers, as demonstrated in a recent study [17]. These parents/caregivers tend to use larger amounts of toothpaste as the baby grows. Also, they tend to use significant variations from the ideal portion, which may interfere with the preventive effect of the dentifrice or have a greater influence on the development of fluorosis. Such observations show the importance of adequate guidance for parents/caregivers, preferably demonstrating the ideal amount with a toothbrush and toothpaste.

3. Fluoride varnishes

In this topic, the use of fluoride varnishes for the prevention of carious lesions and the treatment of initial lesions in enamel is discussed. This is not the first choice of dental material for the treatment of dentin lesions, but it may be considered a good treatment option for enamel lesions, mostly white spot lesions.

According to the American Dental Association (ADA), in addition to silver diamine fluoride (SDF) [18], fluoride varnishes are the only products for professional topical application recommended for use in patients younger than 6 years old [19].

The main advantages of fluoride varnishes are the prolonged contact time with the dental tissue, which favors the absorption of the ion and the formation of calcium fluoride (CaF2) reservoirs, and the possibility of using reduced amounts of the product, minimizing the possibility of ingestion and making it safer for use in babies.

The traditional formulation consists of a natural resin matrix (colophony) with a high concentration of sodium fluoride (22.600 ppm, 2.26% F- ions, or 5% NaF).

The natural resin base forms a film on the tooth surface and, once NaF is exposed to the oral cavity, it dissolves and solubilizes, forming CaF2 reservoirs. The reaction continues for periods up to 24 hours, which is favored by the contact of the varnish with the tooth, because it is time/contact-dependent. Therefore, it is recommended that patients treated with fluoride varnishes remain without brushing their teeth for different periods [20], which can vary from 45 minutes after application to 24 hours. This procedure not only increases the amount of CaF2 formed, but also favors remineralization over time [20].

3.1 Effectiveness of fluoride varnish for prevention and treatment of caries disease in babies

Varnishes can be applied to a specific carious lesion, where they will have a therapeutic/remineralizing effect, or to the entire dentition for a preventive effect.

Analyzing randomized clinical trials that studied the preventive effect of fluoride varnishes applied twice a year, it was observed that, in babies aged 18 to 47 months old, the preventable fraction was 31%, namely, there is 31% more chance that babies who received varnish treatment will not develop caries lesions when compared to those who did not receive the treatment [21]. On the other hand, with the same frequency of application, treatment with varnish in patients aged 2 to 5 years old had a preventive effect similar to supervised toothbrushing [22]. Systematic reviews on this topic are also available. The first one shows that the estimated preventable fraction in patients who received the application of fluoride varnish is 37% (95% CI 25–51%) when compared to placebo or no treatment and, therefore, there is a protective effect in deciduous teeth [9]. The second, considering the same comparison, found a protective effect of varnish on the tooth surface, but with questionable clinical relevance, concluding that the preventive effect of fluoride varnish is uncertain [23]. What is common in both reviews is that primary studies (those studies from which data are extracted) are at high-risk of bias or uncertain bias. Still, the preventive use of fluoride varnishes in babies is recommended by the American Dental Association (ADA) [19, 24] and by the International Association of Pediatric Dentistry [25].

There is consensus in the literature regarding the ability of varnish to remineralize enamel lesions. Among non-restorative treatments, varnish is effective [24, 26], with better results than fluoride gel [27]. In the remineralization of initial carious lesions of deciduous teeth, fluoride varnish with 5% NaF reached the level of 65.9% (95% CI 41.2–90.7%) of inactivated lesions [28]. The remineralizing capacity of varnish was also confirmed when only studies with patients with ECC (early childhood caries) were considered [29].

The vast majority of studies are performed with Duraphat (Colgate-Palmolive), which was the first fluoride varnish manufactured in the 1960s and is considered the gold standard when it comes to research. However, variations have been observed in the formulas of fluoride varnishes, with the addition of active ingredients such as tricalcium phosphate (TCP), calcium and phosphate, calcium sodium phosphosilicate (CSPS), amorphous calcium phosphate (ACP), casein phosphopeptide and amorphous calcium phosphate (CPP-ACP), xylitol, among others [30], aiming to increase the formation of CaF_2 on the tooth surface and potentialize remineralization in the body of the lesion [31], in a synergistic effect with fluorine. Varnishes with 5% NaF and CPP-ACP [32] and with TCP have already demonstrated, in randomized clinical trials, greater remineralizing potential than varnish exclusively based on 5% NaF in children with ECC.

3.2 Application protocol and periodicity

The application of fluoride varnish is indicated for babies with high-risk or caries activity; for low-risk patients who live in regions with fluoridated water, there is no need for professional fluoride application, for these patients, only brushing with fluoridated dentifrice is recommended.

The fluoride varnish application protocol has variations according to the manufacturer's instructions. Some products require humidity for application on tooth surface

Sodium Fluoride-Based Varnishes		
Product	**% of Fluor. Other active components**	**Protocols**
Duraphat (Colgate-Palmolive GmbH, Waltrop, Germany) 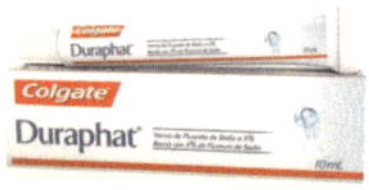	5% Sodium Fluoride	1. Exclusive dentist use. 2. Clean and dry the surface. 3. Apply with a brush in a thin layer on the areas to be treated.
Biophat (Biodinamica, Ibiporá, PR, Brazil) 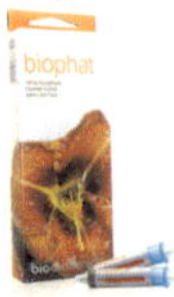	6% Sodium Fluoride	1. Prophylaxis and removal of excess moisture from the teeth. 2. Application with a brush in the desired areas. 3. Patient: do not eat solid food during the first 4 hours; do not brush your teeth 24 hours after application to avoid removing the varnish film prematurely. 4. It is recommended to make 2 to 3 applications with an interval of 3 to 4 days.

Varnishes based on Sodium Fluoride and Calcium Fluoride		
Product	**% of Fluor. Other active components**	**Protocols (by fabricants)**
Duafluond XII (FGM, Joinvile, SC, Brazil) 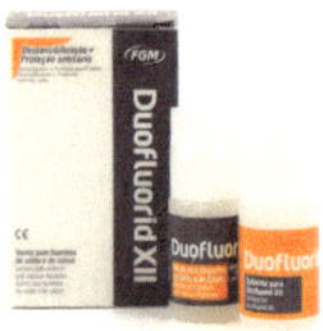	6% Sodium Fluoride 6% Calcium Fluoride	1. Cleaning and drying the surface to be treated; 2. Product homogenization; 3. Application on the surface to be treated; 4. After 10 to 20 seconds, dry with compressed air; 5. Careful brushing for the first 24 h to avoid premature removal of the varnish
Bifluorid 12 (VOCO GmbH, Cuxhaven, Germany) 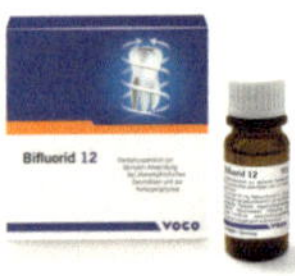	6% Sodium Fluoride 6% Calcium Fluoride	1. Clean and dry the surfaces; 2. Varnish homogenization; 3. Application on surfaces in a thin layer with a brush; 4. Absorption for 10 to 20 seconds and air drying; 5. No toothbrushing for 12 to 24 h after application

Varnishes with other associated active components		
Product	**% of Fluor. Other active components**	**Protocols (by fabricants)**
Mi Varnish (GC. Tokyo, Japan 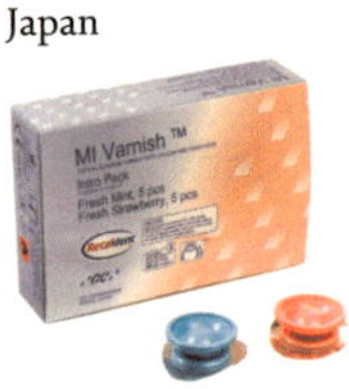	5% Sodium Fluoride CPP-ACP (1–5%)	1. Clean and dry tooth surfaces; 2. Applying a thin, ever layer of varnish to the teeth using a microbrush. If there is separation between the components, homogenize with microbrush; 3. MI Varnish takes prey on contact with water/saliva; 4. Patients: avoid hard, hot or sticky foods, toothbrushing, flossing for 4 h after application.

Varnishes with other associated active components		
Product	**% of Fluor. Other active components**	**Protocols (by fabricants)**
3 M Fast Release Varnish (3 M ESPE Saint Paul, USA) 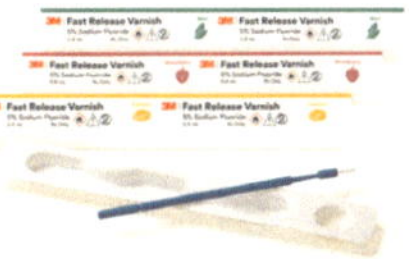	5% Sodium Fluoride Xylitol	1. Dental brushing or prophylaxis and drying of the surfaces to be treated; 2. Opening the single-dose package and mixing the varnish with the applicator provided; 3. Application of the varnish with the applicator, forming a thin layer on the treated area; 4. Patient: do not brush teeth, floss, or consume hot drinks for at least 4 h after treatment.
Clinpro White Varnish (3 M ESPE, Saint Paul, USA) 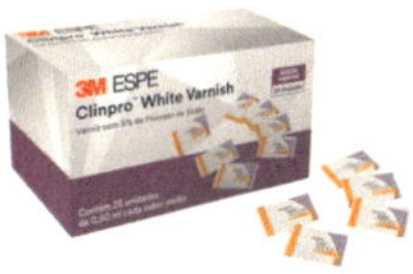	5% Sodium Fluoride 5% Modified Tricalcium Phosphate (TCP)	1. Determining the appropriate dose for the patient (application guide - 0.25 ml - primary dentition); 2. Cleaning the tooth surface (brushing); 3. Mixing the varnish; 4. Application of the product (in the presence of saliva without excess), in a thin layer; 5. Patient: close the mouth to facilitate the setting of the material; 6. Do not rinse or suck immediately after application; 7. Patient: avoid hard and sticky foods, hot drinks, toothbrushing, and flossing for at least 4 h after application.
Fluor Protector (Ivoclar-Vivadent) 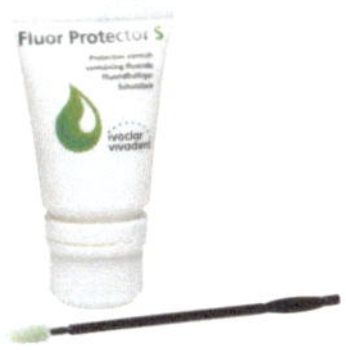	1% Difluorosilane (1.000 ppm F)	1. Dental prophylaxis and relative isolation; 2. Apply a thin layer with a single-use applicator and dental floss (interproximal areas); 3. Disperse and dry the varnish, optionally using an air syringe; 4. Remove insulation after 1 minute; 5. Patient: do not rinse mouth, eat, or brush teeth for 45 minutes.

Table 2.
Commercially available fluoride varnishes, percentage of fluoride, other active components, and protocol of use according to manufacturers.

and others recommend drying the teeth; there are different guidelines regarding the time to restrict toothbrushing and ingestion of hard food after application. Therefore, it is essential to read the instructions before using a specific product. The application characteristics of each varnish, according to the manufacturer's recommendations, is described in **Table 2**.

As for periodicity, it is believed that the preventive effect of fluoride varnish is achieved with 2 to 4 annual applications [9]. The American Dental Association (ADA) recommends the application of varnish every 3–6 months [19, 24], and the International Association of Pediatric Dentistry (IAPD) every 3 months, in patients with high-risk of caries [25].

When fluoride varnish is used for remineralization of initial enamel lesions, there is no standard protocol in the literature. There are reports of two applications (initial consultation and after 4 months), four consecutive weekly applications, applications every 3 months, and even daily applications [27]. More frequent applications can be advantageous, accelerating the inactivation of the carious lesions. Recently, an in vitro study confirmed this hypothesis: the use of fluoride varnish with CPP-ACP applied at 4-week intervals was more effective in remineralizing white spots than applications every 12 or 6 weeks [33]. This effect was observed in permanent teeth, but it can be extrapolated to primary teeth. Therefore, the protocol depends on the individual analysis of the patient, the clinical characteristics of the lesion, and the response obtained during the treatment.

3.3 Toxicity of fluoride varnishes

Even considering the high concentration of fluoride present in varnishes, the possibility of acute toxicity after ingestion of small amounts of the product is practically non-existent. The bioavailability of fluorides was studied after the application of fluoride varnishes in 5-year-old patients, concluding that, despite a transient increase in the amount of fluoride in the urine, the levels returned to normal after 48 hours and the product is safe for use in children [34]. Plasma levels are also far below from the toxic dosage [35].

The probably toxic level of fluoride corresponds to 5 mg of fluoride per kg of body weight. The approximate amount of fluoride in 1 g of fluoride varnish is 22 mg. Approximately 0.5 g of fluoride varnish is used in one application. In order to be toxic, it would be necessary that the baby ingests 4.5 g of varnish at once. Knowing that in a tube of Duraphat (Colgate-Palmolive), the varnish most used in the world, there is 10 mg of the product, the child would have to ingest half of its content at once, which will hardly happen.

The possible adverse effects of using fluoride varnish were evaluated based on 3 different clinical trials carried out with patients with ECC and whose treatment protocol included periodic applications of fluoride varnish. A total of 2.424 children aged between 0 and 5 years old were included. On average, each child received 4 treatments with fluoride varnish. No systemic alterations (nausea, vomiting, etc.) or the need for medical consultation, which could be considered as an adverse effect to the application of fluoride varnish, were reported by parents/guardians within 10 days after treatment. At the end of 3 years of follow-up, no adverse effects were related to the application of fluoride varnish [36].

4. Conclusion

Toothbrushing with fluoridated dentifrice is the main resource to prevent and treat white spot lesions in babies. In patients who are at high-risk of caries and during the active phase of the disease, the association with fluoride varnishes is indicated to accelerate the inactivation process of the lesions. Irrespective of the fluoride treatment selected, when correctly indicated and performed, home-based or professionally applied fluoride treatments are safe for babies and effective in controlling enamel carious lesions.

Conflict of interest

"The authors declare no conflict of interest".

Author details

Ana Cláudia Rodrigues Chibinski*, Anna Bárbara Maluf, Larissa Yumi Ito,
Letícia Maira Wambier, Mayara Vitorino Gevert and Vitória Monteiro
State University of Ponta Grossa, Paraná, Brazil

*Address all correspondence to: anachibinski@hotmail.com; anachibinski@uepg.com

References

[1] Bernabe E, Marcenes W, Hernandez CR, Bailey J, Abreu LG, Alipour V, et al. Global, regional, and National Levels and trends in burden of Oral conditions from 1990 to 2017: A systematic analysis for the global burden of disease 2017 study. Journal of Dental Research. 2020;**99**(4): 362-373

[2] Pitts N, Baez R, Diaz-Guallory C, et al. Early childhood caries: IAPD Bangkok declaration. International Journal of Paediatric Dentistry. 2019;**29**(3):384-386

[3] Uribe SE, Innes N, Maldupa I. The global prevalence of early childhood caries: A systematic review with meta-analysis using the WHO diagnostic criteria. International Journal of Paediatric Dentistry. 2021;**31**(6):817-830

[4] Fejerskov O, Nyvad B, Kidd E. Dental Caries: The Disease and its Clinical Management. 3rd edition. Chichester, West Sussex, UK: John Wiley & Sons Inc.; 2015

[5] Ten Cate JM, Buzalaf MAR. Fluoride mode of action: Once there was an observant dentist. Journal of Dental Research. 2019;**98**(7):725-730

[6] Walsh T, Worthington HV, Glenny AM, Marinho VC, Jeroncic A. Fluoride toothpastes of different concentrations for preventing dental caries. Cochrane Database of Systematic Reviews. 2019;**3** (3):CD007868

[7] Marinho VC, Chong LY, Worthington HV, Walsh T. Fluoride mouthrinses for preventing dental caries in children and adolescents. Cochrane Database of Systematic Reviews. 2016;7(7): CD002284

[8] Marinho VC, Worthington HV, Walsh T, Chong LY. Fluoride gels for preventing dental caries in children and adolescents. Cochrane Database of Systematic Reviews. 2015;**2015**(6): CD002280

[9] Marinho VC, Worthington HV, Walsh T, Clarkson JE. Fluoride varnishes for preventing dental caries in children and adolescents. Cochrane Database of Systematic Reviews. 2013;(7):CD002279

[10] Marinho VC, Higgins JP, Sheiham A, Logan S. Fluoride toothpastes for preventing dental caries in children and adolescents. Cochrane Database of Systematic Reviews. 2003;**2003**(1): CD002278

[11] Cury JA, Tenuta LMA. Riscos do uso do dentifrício fluoretado na prevenção e controle de cárie na primeira infância. Revista da Faculdade de Odontologia de Porto Alegre. 2012;**53**(3):21-27

[12] Wright JT, Hanson N, Ristic H, Whall CW, Estrich CG, Zentz RR. Fluoride toothpaste efficacy and safety in children younger than 6 years: A systematic review. Journal of the American Dental Association (1939). 2014;**145**(2):182-189

[13] Chedid SJ, Tenuta M, Cury JA. O uso de fluoretos em odontopediatria fundamentado em evidências. In: Odontopediatria para o pediatra. Coutinho; Bonecker (coord). São Paulo: Ed.Atheneu; 2013.p. 419-430

[14] Kobayashi CA, Belini MR, Italiani Fde M, Pauleto AR, Araújo JJ, Tessarolli V, et al. Factors influencing fluoride ingestion from dentifrice by children. Community Dentistry and Oral Epidemiology. 2011;**39**(5):426-432

[15] Buzalaf MAR. Review of fluoride intake and appropriateness of current

guidelines. Advances in Dental Research. 2018;**29**(2):157-166

[16] Whelton HP, Spencer AJ, Do LG, Rugg-Gunn AJ. Fluoride revolution and dental caries: Evolution of policies for global use. Journal of Dental Research. 2019;**98**(8):837-846

[17] Coclete GEG, Delbem ACB, Sampaio C, Danelon M, Monteiro DR, Pessan JP. Use of fluoridated dentifrices by children in Araçatuba, Brazil: Factors affecting brushing habits and amount applied on the brush. European Archives of Paediatric Dentistry. 2021;**22**(5): 979-984

[18] Chibinski AC, Wambier LM, Feltrin J, Loguercio AD, Wambier DS, Reis A. Silver diamine fluoride has efficacy in controlling caries progression in primary teeth: A systematic review and meta-analysis. Caries Research. 2017;**51**(5): 527-541

[19] Weyant RJ, Tracy SL, Anselmo TT, Beltrán-Aguilar ED, Donly KJ, Frese WA, et al. Topical fluoride for caries prevention: Executive summary of the updated clinical recommendations and supporting systematic review. Journal of the American Dental Association. 2013; **144**(11):1279-1291

[20] Giacaman R, Fernández C, Muñoz-Sandoval C, Fuentes N. Longer retention time of fluoridated varnishes enhances enamel remineralisation in vitro. Oral Health and Preventive Dentistry. 2017;**15** (6):569-573

[21] Slade GD, Bailie RS, Roberts-Thomson K, Leach AJ, Raye I, Endean C, et al. Effect of health promotion and fluoride varnish on dental caries among Australian Aboriginal children: Results from a community-randomized controlled trial. Community Dentistry and Oral Epidemiology. 2011;**39**(1):29-43

[22] Agouropoulos A, Twetman S, Pandis N, Kavvadia K, Papagiannoulis L. Caries-preventive effectiveness of fluoride varnish as adjunct to oral health promotion and supervised tooth brushing in preschool children: A double-blind randomized controlled trial. Journal of Dentistry. 2014;**42**(10): 1277-1283

[23] de Sousa FSO, Dos Santos APP, Nadanovsky P, Hujoel P, Cunha-Cruz J, de Oliveira BH. Fluoride varnish and dental caries in preschoolers: A systematic review and meta-analysis. Caries Research. 2019;**53**(5):502-513

[24] Slayton RL, Urquhart O, Araujo MW, Fontana M, Guzmán-Armstrong S, Nascimento MM, et al. Evidence-based clinical practice guideline on nonrestorative treatments for carious lesions: A report from the American Dental Association. Journal of the American Dental Association. 2018;**149** (10):837-849

[25] IAPD. Foundational Articles and Consensus Recommendations: Caries Risk Assessment and Care Pathways. 2020

[26] Urquhart O, Tampi MP, Pilcher L, Slayton RL, Araujo MWB, Fontana M, et al. Nonrestorative treatments for caries: Systematic review and network meta-analysis. Journal of Dental Research. 2019;**98**(1):14-26

[27] Lenzi TL, Montagner AF, Soares FZ, de Oliveira RR. Are topical fluorides effective for treating incipient carious lesions?: A systematic review and meta-analysis. Journal of the American Dental Association. 2016;**147**:84-91.e81

[28] Gao SS, Zhang S, Mei ML, Lo EC, Chu CH. Caries remineralisation and arresting effect in children by professionally applied fluoride treatment

- A systematic review. BMC Oral Health. 2016;**16**:12

[29] Schmoeckel J, Gorseta K, Splieth CH, Juric H. How to intervene in the caries process: Early childhood caries - A systematic review. Caries Research. 2020;**54**(2):102-112

[30] Downey D, Dennison J, Eckert GJ, Flannagan SE, Neiva GF, Yaman P, et al. Fluoride levels in unstimulated whole saliva following clinical application of different 5% NaF varnishes. Caries Research. 2018;**52**(6):431-438

[31] Godoi FA, Carlos NR, Bridi EC, Amaral FLBD, França FMG, Turssi CP, et al. Remineralizing effect of commercial fluoride varnishes on artificial enamel lesions. Brazilian Oral Research. 2019;**33**:e044

[32] Radha S, Kayalvizhi G, Adimoulame S, Prathima GS, Muthusamy K, Ezhumalai G, et al. Comparative evaluation of the remineralizing efficacy of fluoride varnish and its combination varnishes on white spot lesions in children with ECC: A randomized clinical trial. International Journal of Clinical Pediatric Dentistry. 2020;**13**(4): 311-317

[33] Abufarwa M, Noureldin A, Campbell PM, Buschang PH. How different time intervals between repeated applications of CPP-ACP fluoride varnish effect smooth surface enamel demineralization? Journal of Dentistry. 2021;**112**:103742

[34] Olympio KP, Cardoso VE, Bijella MF, Pessan JP, Delbem AC, Buzalaf MA. Urinary fluoride output in children following the use of a dual-fluoride varnish formulation. Journal of Applied Oral Science. 2009;**17**(3):179-183

[35] Ekstrand J, Koch G, Petersson LG. Plasma fluoride concentration and urinary fluoride excretion in children following application of the fluoride-containing varnish Duraphat. Caries Research. 1980;**14**(4):185-189

[36] Garcia RI, Gregorich SE, Ramos-Gomez F, Braun PA, Wilson A, Albino J, et al. Absence of fluoride varnish-related adverse events in caries prevention trials in young children, United States. Preventing Chronic Disease. 2017;**14**:E17

Chapter 5

Current Concepts on Caries Removal

Urvashi Bhimjibhai Sodvadia

Abstract

This chapter offers a comprehensive introduction of dental caries management, with a central emphasis on selective caries removal as a cornerstone of minimally invasive dentistry. Rooted in evidence-based dentistry and a grasp of carious dentin progression, the shift from conventional dental paradigms is explored. Various challenges and debates surrounding selective caries removal techniques are discussed, encompassing non-selective, selective, and stepwise methods. Histological and clinical identification methods for carious dentin are explored till the date, including color, hardness, and texture variations. It is important to pay attention to the connection between tactile examinations and the International Caries Detection and Assessment System (ICDAS) index. The relationship between clinical staging and histological aspects of carious dentin is established. Diverse techniques like hand excavation, polymer-based burs, chemomechanical agents, air abrasion, lasers, and tungsten carbide burs are evaluated, highlighting benefits, limitations, and comparisons. The chapter underscores selective caries removal's role in minimally invasive dentistry, focusing on tissue preservation and its impact on pulp vitality, restoration durability, and patient well-being. This comprehensive presentation covers clinical, histological, and technological facets of caries management in a minimally invasive context.

Keywords: contemporary methods, dental caries, demineralized dentin, remineralized dentin, selective caries removal

1. Introduction

Dental caries is the most common dental disease caused by an imbalance between healthy microorganisms and cariogenic species. This ecological shift is developed and maintained by frequent consumption of fermentable dietary carbohydrates. This imbalance might disrupt the demineralization and compensation cycles, resulting in net mineral loss of the tooth structure, which leads to dental cavities [1].

Dental caries cannot be completely cured by only eliminating the causative microorganisms. Instead, it can also be treated by behavioral management. It includes reduction in consumption of fermentable dietary carbohydrates and frequent disruption of bacterial biofilm from the tooth surface. Bacterial penetration cannot be prevented if such management is not being practiced by the patients which can result in irreversible inflammatory damage to the pulp [2].

Contemporary dental practice is based on evidence-based dentistry, a clear understanding of carious dentin progress, and an awareness of potential of remineralizable dentin. Therefore, a shift from G. V. Black's concept of 'extension for prevention' to minimally invasive dentistry is being employed in the clinical practice [3]. Despite the development of adhesive dentistry and spreading awareness of environmental alarms over mercury levels, the acceptance towards minimally invasive techniques for caries removal is debatable. Therefore, Selective Caries Removal in Permanent Teeth (SCRiPT) Trial is being conducted to remove the barrier of confusion on this subject [4].

This chapter emphasizes the importance of selective caries removal approach, highlighting its advantages in preserving tooth structure, pulp vitality, and longevity. Different methods of caries removal, including non-selective, selective, and stepwise techniques, are discussed, with selective removal offering favorable outcomes. Histological analysis assists in distinguishing remineralizable and healthy dentin layers that provide guidance for an accurate excavation. The use of various caries removal techniques like polymer-based burs, chemomechanical agents, air abrasion, lasers, and tungsten carbide burs are explored.

2. Concepts of caries removal

According to a consensus assessment published by Schwendicke et al. numerous approaches of caries eradication have been explained in the literature and can be classified into three types [5]:

- *Non-selective caries removal*: The softened dentine in the cavity is removed until hard dentin is reached throughout the cavity, and the tooth is permanently restored.

- *Selective caries removal:* Caries removal differs depending on the location of the cavity. When all caries has been eliminated, the cavity will have hard dentin around its outer perimeter and soft dentin in the middle of the cavity, which can be readily excavated with a spoon excavator without exposing the pulp. Following that, a permanent restoration is placed at the same appointment.

- *Stepwise caries removal*: This procedure consists of two different sessions scheduled 6–12 months apart. The initial session involves selective caries removal and the temporary restoration of the cavity. In the subsequent visit, the caries is completely removed, and the tooth is restored with a permanent restoration.

Although selective caries removal in a single visit presents more favorable outcome than step-wise selective caries removal approach, this has been remained as a controversy among the dental practitioners [6]. This can be due to inability to compare the long-term outcome between two techniques. One explanation for the preference for one-step selective caries removal is the avoidance of iatrogenic damage to the tooth structure while re-entering the cavity in order to replace the tooth with a permanent restoration, which would have been unavoidable with stepwise caries removal [7].

The primary goal of removing carious lesion is to preserve the pulp vitality in order to increase the tooth longevity in the mouth [8].

Recent recommendation on caries removal by consensus statement by Schwendicke et al. [9]:

- Selective caries removal to firm dentin is advisable for the teeth with shallow or moderate cavity lesion.

- Selective removal to soft dentin is strongly advised for the primary teeth with radiographic evidence of deeper lesion (into pulpal third of the dentin); whereas for permanent teeth with the same criteria, either selective (to soft dentin) or stepwise removal should be performed.

3. What makes selective caries removal the cornerstone of minimally invasive dentistry?

Minimally invasive dentistry focuses on preservation of soft and hard dental tissue when managing carious lesions. This technique not only encompasses removal of carious lesion to firm dentin, but it also includes conservative approach including behavioral modification. This approach comprises of diet modification, disruption of biofilm by chemical or mechanical ways, and cutting of the nutrient supply of cariogenic biofilm by sealing it hermitically [10]. When this principle is applied to the operative dentistry, it can be inferred that selective caries excavation followed by placement of a restoration with hermetic peripheral seal will preserve the dental tissue even without having complete eradication of bacteria from carious dentin.

Traditional non-selective caries removal technique can result in dentin-pulp complex damage, compromised mechanical integrity of tooth structure, and in some cases, it can also lead to irreversible damage primary odontoblasts. Conversely, contemporary selective caries removal can preserve the remineralizable dentinal structure and primary odontoblast that will help in forming tertiary or reactionary dentin [10]. By dropping the burden of cariogenic bacteria, it reduces the number of bacteria approaching pulpal tissue via dentinal tubules. By and large, it boosts the tooth life and decreases management cost and burden associated with teeth overtime [9].

It should be noted that even though the adhesion of composite resin to remineralizable dentin is weaker, it is clinically nonsignificant and cannot hamper the overall outcome of tooth restoration. This can be explained by formation of hermetic seal of resin-based adhesive to peripheral sound enamel or dentin in aptly prepared cavity [11].

The primary challenge with the selective caries removal procedure is the ability to distinguish carious dentin clinically. Sometimes, it becomes difficult to decide the extent of removal, which may impact overall long-term outcome of the restoration.

4. How can we clinically distinguish between different stages of dental caries?

Carious dentin can be identified clinically based on the color, hardness, texture and results of caries detecting dyes. Following part describes the different techniques of caries identification, and their clinical comparison based on the literature.

Among all the techniques, visual and tactile examination are the most commonly employed techniques. The primary dentinal carious lesion can be categorized into four different types when it is examined under natural daylight or standard dental light. These four colors are yellow, light brown, dark brown, and black. Whereas, Hellyer et al. categorized hardness of dentinal carious lesion as hard, medium (leathery), and soft [12].

The hardness of non-carious dentin ranges between 51 and 65 KHN. It drops down to 6.7 KHN in presence of active lesion, whereas hardness of arrested lesion reduces to 39.2 KHN. In other words, hardness of remineralizable and healthy dentin is 30.7 and 60 KHN, respectively [13].

Clinically, the texture or hardness can be evaluated using a new Ash No. 6 prob. The hard lesions are similar to the intact dentin. When moderate pressure is employed, a fresh Ash No. 6 probe can easily penetrate medium or leathery lesions and encounters resistance during withdrawal. Although soft lesions demonstrate smooth penetration of a fresh Ash No. 6 prob. with no resistance upon its withdrawal [14, 15].

The active and inactive carious lesions show different characteristics in terms of color and texture. **Table 1** and **Figure 1** show the difference in signs of staging of carious lesions [16]. The visual and tactile examinations show high specificity but due to subjective nature of tests, they show less reproducibility, and low sensitivity [17].

		Initial and moderate stage	Extensive Stage
Active lesion	color	Whitish/yellowish opaque area	
	Gloss	Loss of luster	
	Hardness and texture	Rough upon probing	Soft and leathery upon probing
	Plaque	Presence of thick plaque	
Arrested lesion	color	Whitish, brownish or black area	
	Gloss	Shiny	
	Hardness and texture	Hard and smooth upon probing	
	Plaque	Absence of plaque	

Table 1.
Outlines clinically identifiable aspects of active and inactive lesions at various stages of cavity lesion progression.

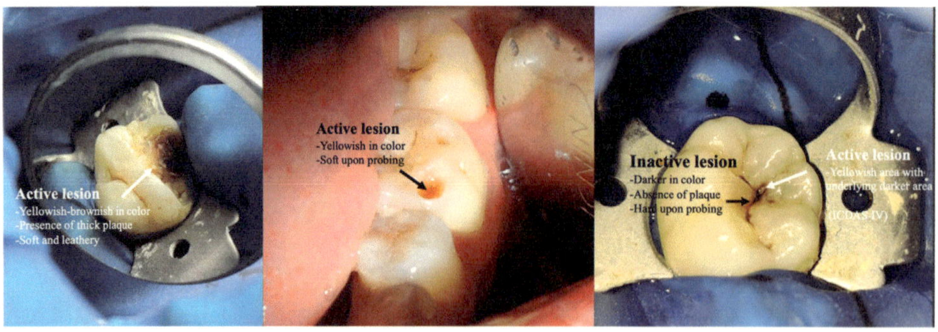

Figure 1.
Three distinct case situations that demonstrate active and inactive lesions depending on certain characteristics. The images on the left and center show active lesions, whereas the image on the right shows a tooth with both types of lesions.

According to the recent systemically reviewed evidences, when we compare the visual and tactile examination, the later produces results with more reliability and specificity. Therefore, it is desirable to opt for the tactile examination over the visual inspection when performing routine inspections to identify caries. It could be stated that texture variations warrant a higher index score. This evidence is in accordance to the current recommended dental caries scoring index, the International and Caries Detection Assessment System (ICDAS) [18].

5. How is the clinical categorization of stages connected to the histological characteristics of dentinal caries?

In the literature, correlation between different color, hardness, and texture of the carious dentin to histological staging of the carious process has been described. The clinical changes of the carious lesion can be resulted from the acidic attack of the cariogenic microorganisms. This acidic dissolution can change the color, texture, and the moisture element of dentinal tissue. Based on the color and texture of the dentinal tissue, the histological staging can be discriminated [19].

To identify the clinical carious examination technique with high sensitivity and specificity, it is advisable to compare the available methods in relation to the microbial activities in form of CFU. This will enable us to identify an accurate consistent method to evaluate caries quantitatively and qualitatively [18].

There are a few research that investigated the relationship between bacterial CFU and the color or hardness of carious dentin in the literature. Orhan et al. found no significant difference in bacteria CFU and color of carious dentin, although harder lesions had considerably fewer bacteria CFU than softer dentin [20]. Comparable outcomes were noted in the Lynch et al. investigation. They discovered that soft and leathery lesions, regardless of color, had greater CFU. There was no association between the color of the lesion and the overall number of bacterial species [21].

6. Which portion of the dentinal caries needs to be eliminated during the selective caries removal?

The precise point at which caries excavation ends clinically is ambiguous and remains subjective. As a particular dentist may be influenced by their own personal experiences, diagnostic tests such as surface hardness, dentin color, or caries detector dyes, are not completely reliable. As a result, a histological analysis is the optimal tool for evaluating carious changes in the dentin and obtaining consistent results to evaluate excavation procedures.

It has been observed that the carious dentin can be divided into distinctive layers using histological staining such as outer dentin containing non-remineralizable necrotic collagen matrix and cariogenic bacteria, and inner layer composed of non-altered collagen fibers. The bacterial count is negligible in the inner layer, and the possibility of remineralization is higher [22].

Mallory-Azan staining allow to differentiate histological staging of carious dentin. Blue staining is identified as un-denatured collagen containing dentin; while altered collagen matrix will catch red staining. Thus, clinically it enables accurate identification of remineralizable or healthy dentin and demineralized dentin, respectively [23].

As previously mentioned in the chapter, hardness is a better ____ to evaluate the severity of carious lesion and plays an important role in determining treatment modalities as well. For instance, softer lesion needs the immediate intrusive clinical modality (e.g., debridement and restoration) as it harbors more cariogenic microorganisms as compare to the harder lesions which does not contain any cariogenic microorganisms. Therefore, harder shallow lesion does not demand any clinical interventions [14].

Selective carious removal to firm dentin is advisable for moderately deep active areas. This procedure allows leathery dentin to left behind at the center of cavity towards pulpal area, whereas caries should be removed until firm hard dentin is reached towards the peripheral dentin and marginal walls of the cavity. Clinical terminology refers to leathery dentine as having a small "tackiness" and not deforming when an object is placed against it. Hard dentine requires pushing pressure to engage, and a scratchy sound known as "cri dentinaire" can be heard [3].

7. What is the recommended method for removing dental caries?

The traditional approach of treating dental caries entails removing the remineralizable tooth tissue and replacing it with a restorative substance. Using a dental air rotor drill is currently the most popular way to remove cavities. Despite its extensive use, potential side effects include dentinal sensitivity, intense noises while using, thermal stimulation of the pulpal tissue, bone-conducted vibration, and pressure inside the tooth itself. Whereas hand excavation allows the operator to have tactile sensation while removing carious tissue. Rotary instruments greatly limit tactile feedback during selective excavation and increase the possibility of iatrogenic removal of extra tooth structure at this critical region [24]. Other techniques investigated include air abrasion, chemical agents, polymer burs, and lasers for the eradication of caries.

7.1 Tungsten carbide bur

Utilizing burs on a high-speed handpiece to reach the carious area and a low-speed handpiece to eliminate carious dentine are the most common approaches for removing caries and preparing cavities. Steel bur excavation and traditional rotary practices result in over-preparation by removing greatest amount of sound tissue possible while potentially overextending the cavity and destroying healthy tissue. Additionally, it generates pressure and heat on the pulp, vibration, noise, causes pain stimulus, and requires the need for local anesthetic. This approach leaves aversion and pain anxiety in many individuals, particularly children [25].

Studies have been conducted to compare the traditional approach with other techniques. Divya et al. investigated the time required to remove the caries and found that the traditional burs (151 sec) remove caries faster as compared to Polymer bur (344.80 sec), Papacarie (359.60 sec), and Carisolv (461.60 sec). The number of bacterial colonies after caries excavation differed considerably among the four agents utilized, with Polymer bur samples containing the highest and Stainless Steel Bur representing only 10% of the specimens [26]. Whereas Somani et al. found no significant difference in the presence of microorganisms following caries eradication between traditional burs and smart burs [27].

7.2 Polymer based bur

The fundamental objective behind developing a polymer-based bur was to create a device with a hardness of 40–50 KHN, which falls between the hardness of healthy and cariously infected dentin. As a result, they selectively remove demineralized dentin and whenever the cutting edges come into touch with either healthy or remineralizable dentin, they become blunted. **Table 2** described characteristics and specifications of available the polymer based burs and traditional carbide bur.

There was no significant difference in the outcome was observed by Usha and Ranjani when different types of polymer bur were compared [28]. Furthermore, Lohmann in et al. concluded that PolyBur P1 was only able to remove carious dentin from 33.9% of the carious teeth specimen. Additionally, the remaining denatured collagen layer was significantly thicker (more than 1 mm) than in the conventional carbide bur group [13].

7.3 Chemomechanical caries removal agents (CMCR)

Since 1975, this modality has been utilized to soften diseased dentin before carefully removing it with hand devices. Because it only affects demineralized dentin, the goal of conserving damaged dentin can be achieved [29]. They are classified into two types: sodium hypochlorite (NaOCl)-based agents (e.g. GK-101, GK-101e, Carisolv) and enzyme-based agents (Papacarie, Biosolv, Carie-Care, Brix3000).

By subsequently destroying the irreparably weakened collagen fibers in demineralized dentin, CMCR chemicals enable removal while preserving the remaining intact impacted dentin [30]. Chlorination, which entails hydrolysis of linkages between tropocollagen components and/or breaking of polypeptide chains in the triple helix, is the key technique used to do this [31]. However, little is yet known about the chemistry of amino acid chlorination and its effects. In contrast to enzyme-based CMCR agents, which rely on an additional mechanism, NaOCl-based CMCR products use the chlorination process as their main mode of action [32].

The fundamental mode of action in enzyme-based CMCR agents is papain, which is considered an effective chemical debriding agent with antibacterial and anti-inflammatory properties. It is a cysteine protease developed from the fruits and latex of green papaya (Carica papaya. The papain is believed to work by promoting the decomposition of partially deteriorated collagen strands and assisting in the deconstruction and removal of fibrin mantle created by carious process and causing no harm to unaffected collagen filaments. As a result, the demineralized dentin softens, making it possible to remove it with no anesthesia and using non-cutting instruments. An absence of –1-antitrypsin in demineralized dentin rationalizes such unique relationship [33].

A risk to dental practitioners' wellbeing exists during the COVID-19 pandemic because many dental treatments generate aerosols that could be associated with the transmission of serious respiratory illnesses. Consequently, dental and health professionals cautioned against overusing aerosol-generating therapies during the outbreak. Given the aforementioned suggestions, utilizing CMCR products that need little to no aerosol-generating techniques instead of surgery in caries prevention may be more proficient for people of all ages, especially those who suffer from anxiety or have special needs [34].

The CMCR approach is becoming more commonly recognized and comfortable for patients, as it reduces pain, anxiety, and the need for a local anesthetic. Hosein

Bur type	Specifications	Hardness	Recommended speed	Specifications
Conventional carbide bur	Tungsten carbide	1600 KHN	1250 rpm–5000 rpm	—
SmartP (2003)	Polyether-ketonne-ketone (PEKK)	50 KHN	500 rpm–800 rpm	First polymer bur
SmartBur II	Glass-bead reinforced blades	50 KHN	5000 rpm–10,000 rpm	Available in three different sizes (#4, #6, and #8) Remove decay in a circular motion, starts from the center and proceed to the periphery. Reduce the contact with axial walls
PolyBur P1	Reinforced polymer	40–50 KHN	2000 rpm - 8000 rpm	Recommended for small cavities, and area close to the pulp Delicate shaft design, more contact pressure tends to bend the shaft No rounding of cutting edges Contraindicated for dark demineralized dentin, hard mineralizable dentin, and caries along the enamel-dentin junction

Table 2.
Describes the available polymer-based burs and conventional carbide burs along with their properties and specifications.

and Hasan reported the procedural time for CMCR as 12.97 min in 27 cases, whereas convention steel bur took 7.4 min for caries removal [35]. The CMCR approach could be taken into account as a possible replacement therapy modality in the field of dental care in the future, despite its extended length and greater expense.

7.4 Air abrasion

Air abrasion, utilized as a method for removing caries, involves the non-rotary abrading of a surface by directing a stream of high-speed abrasive particles produced from compressed air. Its mechanism involves cutting at the tip and shapes shallow, saucer-like cavities with vague boundaries. In contrast to rotary drilling, air abrasion's use of extremely small particles in contact with the tooth prevents the generation of vibrational forces, resulting in enhanced comfort and reduced stress on the tooth structure. This is especially beneficial in the dentine area near the pulp, where delicate caries elimination using the slow-speed handpiece is often uncomfortable due to the resulting vibrations. In this context, employing air abrasion with a slow cutting action becomes a practical choice. The forceful expulsion of particles through the air stream also reduces the effort required by the operator [36].

Aluminum oxide abrasives are commonly used for air abrasion in dentistry, but concerns exist regarding their potential to damage healthy tooth structure and controversial safety issues [37]. An alternative option is bioactive glass (Sylc), initially designed for bone replacement. Sylc, a bioactive glass abrasive, is available for tooth polishing and has shown potential for selective cutting. However, its cutting time is significantly longer than alumina, making it less practical [38].

Neither alumina nor Sylc contains fluoride, despite evidence of fluoride-assisted remineralization in dentine.

Farooq et al. have explored fluoride-incorporated bioactive glass, discovering that reducing sodium content increases its hardness, which could be advantageous for creating bioactive glass air abrasives. Additionally, they demonstrated apatite formation in bioactive glass in Tris buffer solution, with potential implications for its abrasiveness compared to alumina in dentine air abrasion [39]. Tan et al. invented a new customized fluoridated bioactive glass particles (Na0SR) and compared its efficacy against standard aluminum oxide particles. It was concluded that Na0SR can be considered a viable abrasive alternative for alumina in air abrasion cutting because it performs similarly and has the added benefit of potentially facilitating remineralization and hydroxyfluorapatite production [40].

7.5 Lasers

The initial dental lasers (ruby, Nd:YAG, holmium-doped Ho:YAG, CO_2 lasers) led to elevated pulp temperature, microcracks, and carbonization. In the mid-1990s, the safety and effectiveness of erbium-doped Er:YAG laser were explored. Proper settings and water cooling minimized thermal damage [41]. Effective caries removal requires a laser wavelength that interacts significantly with mineral, water, or both, unless ultrashort pulses cause plasma-mediated ablation.

Er:YAG and erbium: yttrium-scandium-gallium-garnet Er:YSGG lasers (λ = 2.940 μm and λ = 2.790 μm) are highly absorbed by water and Er:YSGG is also absorbed by hydroxyl ions in tooth mineral, heating and exploding tissue from the surface. For effective caries removal, the laser pulse duration should approximately match the tissue's "thermal relaxation time," avoiding excessively short or long pulse durations that result in excessive or unnecessary energy distribution within the tissue [42]. The Food and Drug Administration (FDA) granted approval for its use in these applications in May 1997. This laser functions in a pulsed manner and incorporates a water spray in its handpiece to prevent tissue dryness and the accumulation of heat. This ensures efficient absorption of energy without causing tissue carbonization or significant heat production [43].

Montedori et al. conducted a systematic review and found no studies reported presence of residual caries after using laser to remove primary caries [44]. In a study conducted by Lui et al.; patients reported limited incidence of pain in Er:YAG laser group than drill group [45].

The carbon dioxide laser lasers can function within the wavelength range of 9000 to 11,000 nm. The most prevalent variant, working at 10,600 nm, is commonly utilized for dental procedures. This laser enables surgical operations without bleeding and minimizes discomfort following soft tissue dental surgeries. Investigations demonstrated that a 9300 nm carbon dioxide laser can prompt both chemical and structural alterations in hard dental tissues [46]. Moreover, it was observed that this laser efficiently eradicates enamel and dentine. Due to its capacity to prevent enamel cavities and eliminate caries lesions, the 9300 nm carbon dioxide laser is gaining increased attention in the field of dentistry for managing dental caries [47].

For laser treatment, the increase in pulp chamber temperature should not be greater than 5.5°C. Otherwise, severe heat buildup could harm the dentine-pulp complex by disrupting odontoblasts, destroying them, or possibly causing pulp necrosis. According to a series of studies, the thermal effect of 9300 nm carbon dioxide laser irradiation on pulp is minimal because the laser is absorbed extremely close to the surface of the hard tissues and shortly converted into heat [48]. Assa et al. also reported that the usage of water aerosol spray with laser would significantly decreases the heat accumulation.

Exposure of enamel to a 9300 nm carbon dioxide laser leads to decomposition of its constituents. This process can cause enamel to melt and fuse due to the temporary elevation in temperature, which exceeds a certain threshold. The laser modifies the enamel's microstructure and surface appearance after it cools down. Additionally, the laser induces chemical transformations in dental hard tissues, including a reduction in carbonate levels. This change transforms carbonated apatite crystals into purer forms, rendering enamel less susceptible to acid erosion. Moreover, the calcium and phosphorus content in both enamel and dentine increases following laser treatment. The dentine subjected to irradiation displays three distinct intrinsic phosphate bands under Fourier transform infrared microscopy, indicating heightened crystallinity. A study highlights that the 9300 nm carbon dioxide laser raises the calcium-phosphorus ratio in healthy enamel and dentine, thus reducing their solubility. Furthermore, the results imply that the laser treatment eliminates organic components from decayed enamel and dentine [49].

8. What factors contribute to a favorable prognosis for the selective caries removal method?

A growing database of studies has also demonstrated that the selective caries excavation technique is prognostically effective. This procedure avoids injuring the dentine-pulp complex and removing a significant quantity of tooth tissue, preserving the pulp's vitality and improving the tooth's long-term prognosis.

In the management of deep carious lesions, it's essential to thoroughly assess the final restoration to prevent potential failures in the tooth-restorative complex. Dentists should carefully inspect the restoration for surface irregularities and proper marginal integrity to avoid creating areas where plaque can accumulate. Leaving some carious tissue under a restoration after selective excavation could lead to legal issues. Patients need to be informed about the rationale behind this approach and the need for regular check-ups to ensure the tooth's pulp health over time Nevertheless, for long-term stability, cuspal coverage would be necessary to counteract the impact of repeated stress on the restoration for some cases.

9. Conclusion

In conclusion, dental caries, a prevalent condition resulting from an imbalance in oral microorganisms triggered by fermentable carbohydrates, causes mineral loss in tooth structures. Traditional treatment approaches, involving complete bacterial eradication, have shifted towards minimally invasive strategies. Selective caries removal, a pivotal aspect of minimally invasive dentistry, preserves remineralizable dentin, vital odontoblasts, and supports the formation of reactionary dentin. Techniques like polymer-based burs, chemomechanical agents, air abrasion, and lasers offer less discomfort, reduced bacterial count, and more conservative excavation. Clinical staging, utilizing color, hardness, and texture evaluations, assists in precise diagnosis and treatment planning. While challenges persist, evidence supports the effectiveness of selective caries removal, enhancing tooth longevity and patient comfort.

Conflict of interest

The authors declare no conflict of interest.

Author details

Urvashi Bhimjibhai Sodvadia
Nova Southeastern University, Clearwater, Florida, United States

*Address all correspondence to: urvashisodvadiya@gmail.com

References

[1] Fejerskov O, Nyvad B, Kidd EAM, editors. Dental Caries: The Disease and Its Clinical Management. Third edition. John Wiley & Sons Inc.; 2015

[2] Bjørndal L, Ricucci D. Pulp inflammation: From the reversible inflammation to pulp necrosis during caries progression. In: Goldberg M, editor. The Dental Pulp Biology, Pathology, and Regenerative Therapies. Berlin, Germany: Springer; 2014. pp. 125-139. DOI: 10.1007/978-3-642-55160-4_9

[3] Banerjee A, Frencken JE, Schwendicke F, Innes NPT. Contemporary operative caries management: Consensus recommendations on minimally invasive caries removal. British Dental Journal. 2017;**223**:215-222. DOI: 10.1038/sj.bdj.2017.672

[4] Clarkson JE, Ramsay CR, Ricketts D, et al. Selective caries removal in permanent teeth (SCRiPT) for the treatment of deep carious lesions: A randomised controlled clinical trial in primary care. BMC Oral Health. 2021;**21**:336. DOI: 10.1186/s12903-021-01637-6

[5] Schwendicke F, Frencken JE, Bjørndal L, et al. Managing carious lesions. Advances in Dental Research. 2016;**28**:58-67. DOI: 10.1177/002203451663927

[6] Maltz M, Garcia R, Jardim JJ, et al. Randomized trial of partial vs. stepwise caries removal: 3-year follow-up. Journal of Dental Research. 2012;**91**:1026-1031. DOI: 10.1177/0022034512460403

[7] European Society of Endodontology (ESE) developed by, Duncan HF, Galler KM, Tomson PL, et al. European Society of Endodontology position statement: Management of deep caries and the exposed pulp. International Endodontic Journal. 2019;**52**:923-934. DOI: 10.1111/iej.13080

[8] Byers MR, Närhi MVO, Mecifi KB. Acute and chronic reactions of dental sensory nerve fibers to cavities and desiccation in rat molars. The Anatomical Record. 1988;**221**:872-883. DOI: 10.1002/ar.1092210412

[9] Schwendicke F, Frencken JE, Bjørndal L, Maltz M, Manton DJ, Ricketts D, et al. Managing carious lesions: Consensus recommendations on carious tissue removal. Advances in Dental Research. 2016;**28**(2):58-67. DOI: 10.1177/0022034516639271

[10] Banerjee A, Watson TF. Pickard's Guide to Minimally Invasive Operative Dentistry. 10th ed. Oxford: Oxford University Press; 2015. DOI: 10.1038/sj.bdj.2015.878

[11] Yoshiyama M, Tay FR, Doi J, et al. Bonding of self-etch and total-etch adhesives to carious dentin. Journal of Dental Research. 2002;**81**:556-560. DOI: 10.1177/154405910208100811

[12] Hellyer PH, Beighton D, Heath MR, Lynch EJ. Root caries in older people attending a general dental practice in East Sussex. British Dental Journal. 1990;**169**:201-206. DOI: 10.1038/sj.bdj.4807326

[13] Lohmann J, Schäfer E, Dammaschke T. Histological determination of cariously altered collagen after dentin caries excavation with the polymer bur PolyBur P1 in comparison to a conventional bud bur.

Head & Face Medicine. 2019;**15**:1-7. DOI: 10.1186/s13005-019-0205-9

[14] Beighton D, Lynch E, Heath MR. A microbiological study of primary root-caries lesions with different treatment needs. Journal of Dental Research. 1993;**72**:623-629. DOI: 10.1177/00220345930720031201

[15] Chong MJ, Seow WK, Purdie DM, Cheng E, Wan V. Visual-tactile examination compared with conventional radiography, digital radiography, and diagnodent in the diagnosis of occlusal occult caries in extracted premolars. Pediatric Dentistry. 2003;**25**:341-349. Available from: https://pubmed.ncbi.nlm.nih.gov/13678099/

[16] Ismail AI, Pitts NB, Tellez M. The international caries classification and management system (ICCMS™) an example of a caries management pathway. BMC Oral Health. 2015;**15**(1):1-13. DOI: 10.1186/1472-6831-15-S1-S9

[17] Bader JD, Shugars DA, Bonito AJ. A systematic review of the performance of methods for identifying carious lesions. Journal of Public Health Dentistry. 2002;**62**:201-213. DOI: 10.1111/j.1752-7325.2002.tb03446.x

[18] Hon L, Mohamed A, Lynch E. Reliability of colour and hardness clinical examinations in detecting dentine caries severity: A systematic review and meta-analysis. Scientific Reports. 2019;**9**(1):6533. DOI: 10.1038/s41598-019-41270-6

[19] Bjorndal L, Larsen T, Thylstrup A. A clinical and microbiological study of deep carious lesions during stepwise excavation using long treatment intervals. Caries Research. 1997;**31**:411-417. DOI: 10.1159/000262431

[20] Orhan AI, Oz FT, Ozcelik B, Orhan K. A clinical and microbiological comparative study of deep carious lesion treatment in deciduous and young permanent molars. Clinical Oral Investigations. 2008;**12**:369-378. DOI: 10.1007/s00784-008-0208-6

[21] Lynch E, Beighton D. A comparison of primary root caries lesions classified according to colour. Caries Research. 1994;**28**:233-239. DOI: 10.1159/000261971

[22] Kuboki Y, Ohgushi K, Fusayama T. Collagen biochemistry of two layers of carious dentin. Journal of Dental Research. 1977;**56**:1233-1237. DOI: 10.1177/00220345770560102301

[23] Ohgushi K. Collagen fibers in the two layers of carious dentin. 1. Histochemical study. Kōkūbyō Gakkai Zasshi. 1973;**40**:65-74. Available from: https://pubmed.ncbi.nlm.nih.gov/4519994/

[24] Lim ZE, Duncan HF, Moorthy A, McReynolds D. Minimally invasive selective caries removal: A clinical guide. British Dental Journal. 2023;**234**(4):233-240. DOI: 10.1038/s41415-023-5515-4

[25] Celiberti P, Francescut P, Lussi A. Performance of four dentine excavation methods in deciduous teeth. Caries Research. 2006;**40**(2):117-123. DOI: 10.1159/000091057

[26] Divya G, Prasad MG, Vasa AA, Vasanthi D, Ramanarayana B, Mynampati P. Evaluation of the efficacy of caries removal using polymer bur, stainless steel bur, Carisolv, Papacarie–an in vitro comparative study. Journal of Clinical and Diagnostic Research: JCDR. 2015;**9**(7):ZC42. DOI: 10.7860/JCDR/2015/12705.6202

[27] Somani R, Chaudhary R, Jaidka S, Singh DJ. Comparative microbiological

evaluation after caries removal by various burs. International Journal of Clinical Pediatric Dentistry. 2019;**12**(6):524. DOI: 10.5005/jp-journals-10005-1678

[28] Usha C, Ranjani R. Comparative evaluation of two commercially available polymer burs for their efficacy on dentinal caries removal – Split tooth study using polarized light microscopy. Journal of Dental Sciences. 2012;**2**:66-69. DOI: 10.5005/jsd-2-2-66

[29] Hamama HH, Yiu C, Burrow M. Current update of chemomechanical caries removal methods. Australian Dental Journal. 2014;**59**(4):446-456. DOI: 10.1111/adj.12214

[30] Soni HK, Sharma A, Sood PB. A comparative clinical study of various methods of caries removal in children. European Archives of Paediatric Dentistry. 2015;**16**:19-26. DOI: 10.1007/s40368-014-0140-1

[31] Chatterjee AN, Das L, Khushboo B, Saha S, Sarkar S. Chemomechanical caries removal with respect to COVID-19 in dentistry. International Journal of Research and Review. 2020;**7**:517-523. DOI: 10.52403/ijrr

[32] Maragakis GM, Hahn P, Hellwig E. Chemomechanical caries removal: A comprehensive review of the literature. International Dental Journal. 2001;**51**(4):291-299. DOI: 10.1002/j.1875-595x.2001.tb00841.x

[33] Jain K, Bardia A, Geetha S, Goel A. Papacarie: A chemomechanical caries removal agent. IJSS Case Reports Review. 2015;**1**(9):57-60. DOI: 10.17354/cr/2015/33

[34] Souza TF, Martins ML, Magno MB, Vicente-Gomila JM, Fonseca-Gonçalves A, Maia LC. Worldwide research trends on the use of chemical–mechanical caries removal products over the years: A critical review. European Archives of Paediatric Dentistry. 2022;**23**(6):869-883. DOI: 10.1007/s40368-022-00726-6

[35] Hosein T, Hasan A. Efficacy of chemo-mechanical caries removal with Carisolv. Journal of the College of Physicians and Surgeons–Pakistan. 2008;**18**(4):222-225. Available from: https://pubmed.ncbi.nlm.nih.gov/18474155/

[36] Black RB. Airbrasive: Some fundamentals. The Journal of the American Dental Association. 1950;**41**(6):701-710. DOI: 10.14219/jada.archive.1950.0247

[37] Wright GZ, Hatibovic-Kofman S, Millenaar DW, Braverman I. The safety and efficacy of treatment with air abrasion technology. International Journal of Paediatric Dentistry. 1999;**9**(2):133-140. DOI: 10.1046/j.1365-263x.1999.00103.x

[38] Milly H, Austin RS, Thompson I, Banerjee A. In vitro effect of air-abrasion operating parameters on dynamic cutting characteristics of alumina and bio-active glass powders. Operative Dentistry. 2014;**39**(1):81-89. DOI: 10.2341/12-466-L

[39] Farooq I, Tylkowski M, Müller S, Janicki T, Brauer DS, Hill RG. Influence of sodium content on the properties of bioactive glasses for use in air abrasion. Biomedical Materials. 2013;**8**(6):065008. DOI: 10.1088/1748-6041/8/6/065008

[40] Tan MH, Hill RG, Anderson P. Comparing the air abrasion cutting efficacy of dentine using a fluoride-containing bioactive glass versus an alumina abrasive: An in vitro study. International Journal of Dentistry. 2015;**2015**:521901. DOI: 10.1155/2015/521901

[41] Li ZZ, Code JE, Van de Merwe WP. Er: YAG laser ablation of enamel and dentin of human teeth: Determination of ablation rates at various fluences and pulse repetition rates. Lasers in Surgery and Medicine. 1992;**12**(6):625-630. DOI: 10.1002/lsm.1900120610

[42] Featherstone JD, Fried D. Fundamental interactions of laserswith dental hard tissues. Medical Laser Application. 2001;**16**(3):181-194. DOI: 10.1078/1615-1615-00022

[43] Marcelino GD, Lopes JH, Faraoni JJ, Dias PC. The use of Er: YAG laser for dental caries removal. Stomatology Edu Journal. 2021;**8**(3):173-183. DOI: 10.25241/stomaeduj.2021.8(3).art.3

[44] Montedori A, Abraha I, Orso M, D'Errico PG, Pagano S, Lombardo G. Lasers for caries removal in deciduous and permanent teeth. Cochrane Database of Systematic Reviews. 2016;**9**:CD010229. DOI: 10.1002/14651858.CD010229.pub2

[45] Liu JF, Lai YL, Shu WY, Lee SY. Acceptance and efficiency of Er: YAG laser for cavity preparation in children. Photomedicine and Laser Therapy. 2006;**24**(4):489. DOI: 10.1089/pho.2006.24.489

[46] Fried D, Zuerlein MJ, Le CQ, Featherstone JD. Thermal and chemical modification of dentin by 9-11-μm CO2 laser pulses of 5-100-μs duration. Lasers in Surgery and Medicine. 2002;**31**(4): 275-282. DOI: 10.1002/lsm.10100

[47] Rechmann P, Rechmann BM, Groves WH Jr, Le CQ, Rapozo-Hilo ML, Kinsel R, et al. Caries inhibition with a CO_2 9.3 μm laser: An in vitro study. Lasers in Surgery and Medicine. 2016;**48**(5):546-554. DOI: 10.1002/lsm.22497

[48] Assa S, Meyer S, Fried D. Ablation of dental hard tissues with a microsecond pulsed carbon dioxide laser operating at 9.3-μm with an integrated scanner. In: Lasers in Dentistry XIV. Vol. 6843. Issue 684308. 2008. pp. 47-53

[49] Takahashi K, Kimura Y, Matsumoto K. Morphological and atomic analytical changes after CO_2 laser irradiation emitted at 9.3 μm on human dental hard tissues. Journal of Clinical Laser Medicine & Surgery. 1998;**16**(3):167-173. DOI: 10.1089/clm.1998.16.167

Chapter 6

Perspective Chapter: Cost-Effectiveness of Caries Preventive Programs

Thomas Davidson

Abstract

This chapter presents the methodology of health economic evaluations within the field of oral health and more specifically discusses the need for cost-effectiveness analyses of various caries preventive programs. It also deals with prioritized questions of limited resources and effective implementation of caries preventive technologies. As the societal cost of caries preventive interventions may not equal the direct cost of the intervention, the cost-effectiveness results depend also on the perspective and time-horizon of the analysis, and several such key issues are presented. The chapter also presents some basics about simulation modeling techniques and how to deal with uncertainty in health economic evaluations. An example of a cost-effectiveness analysis of a caries preventive program and aspects to consider is furthermore provided, to guide in the economic evaluation. Some evidences of the cost-effectiveness of various caries preventive programs are presented. However, there are some methodological weaknesses in many of the studies, and more research is needed to determine the value of such programs.

Keywords: economic evaluation, cost effectiveness, quality of life, QALY, willingness to pay

1. Introduction

Oral diseases have a significant impact on the global economy, resulting in a burden of over US$700 billion, which includes both direct and indirect costs [1]. This amounts to almost 5% of the global health expenditure. Dental caries is responsible for 15% of this burden, but the actual percentage may be higher due to its association with other oral diseases [2]. Consequently, dental caries presents substantial economic challenges for individuals and healthcare systems alike.

At the same time, dental caries can result in significant health losses, from physical pain and tooth loss to psychological and financial burdens. Hence, there are many reasons to prevent dental caries.

Reducing the incidence of dental caries may be achieved through various programs. However, implementation of these programs requires investment of resources, both private and public. As resources are limited, it is essential to allocate them judiciously. Prioritizing the allocation of resources based on criteria such as effectiveness, ethics, and cost-effectiveness is important.

Comprehensive health economic evaluations play a crucial role in prioritizing healthcare services. Although a significant portion of oral health services is privately paid, there is still a need for guidance in the cost-effective use of resources. Many countries subsidize dentistry to some extent, and it is important that public resources are used efficiently. Moreover, public dental health programs may require health economic evaluations as they involve societal investments.

Health economic evaluations provide decision-makers with valuable information to allocate resources efficiently, develop guidelines, and fund research. They can also identify potential disparities in access to preventive care and oral health outcomes across different population groups. Decision-makers can use this information to direct certain programs to vulnerable groups to improve overall oral health equity.

This chapter presents health economic evaluations, different types of analyses, and some methodological issues such as the perspective and time horizon of the analysis. It briefly explains how to calculate the costs and outcomes of a program, how cost-effectiveness should be understood and interpreted, and the need for simulation studies and uncertainty analyses. A fictive example about the cost-effectiveness of a fluoride varnishing program in school is also presented. Finally, some general findings about the cost-effectiveness of caries preventive programs are discussed.

2. Health economic evaluations

2.1 Type of analyses

When it comes to health economic evaluations, there are various types of analyses. The main difference between them is how the outcomes are handled. In general, all analyses aim to determine the opportunity cost of a particular healthcare program in relation to its additional effects. Opportunity cost refers to the benefits that resources could have yielded if spent in the most optimal way. To determine the opportunity cost of a program, it should be compared with the best alternative [3].

Commonly used health economic analyses are:

- Cost analysis (CA)
- Cost-minimization analysis (CMA)
- Cost-effectiveness analysis (CEA)
- Cost-utility analysis (CUA)
- Cost-benefit analysis (CBA)
- Budget impact analysis (BI)

A cost analysis is a type of evaluation that focuses only on measuring the costs of a program and is not intended to be used for comparing different programs. It does not require a comparator since its purpose is only to determine the cost of a particular program.

A cost-minimization analysis, on the other hand, can be used for prioritizing between different programs. This type of analysis assumes that the consequences of the compared programs are identical. Therefore, it studies the costs of at least two programs and recommends the one with the lowest cost. Ideally, there should be evidence supporting the assumption of equal outcomes to use this analysis; otherwise, it may lead to unintentional rationing.

A cost-effectiveness analysis is used when the outcomes are expected to differ. The outcome measure in such an analysis could be any measure that is relevant to the treatment analyzed, such as life-years gained, the number of infections, prevented decayed, missing, or filled teeth (DMFT), and so on.

A cost-utility analysis is similar to a cost-effectiveness analysis, but it relates outcomes to some kind of values that represent utility or quality of life (QoL), most often quality-adjusted life-years (QALYs).

Another type of analysis is the cost-benefit analysis, which uses monetary terms for both the costs and the outcomes. This is often measured by studying the willingness to pay. If the outcomes are valued higher than the costs in such an analysis, this means that the treatment has a positive net benefit and, hence, that it should be implemented. Such monetary outcomes may be especially relevant in dental care, as people are generally used to paying most of the costs themselves, in contrast to other healthcare fields where much of the cost is often covered by society or insurance companies.

The analyses presented above can be complemented by a budget impact analysis [4], which evaluates how the introduction of a new program affects one or several budgets and what other consequences are expected for the main actors. All types of health economic analyses may be suitable for economic evaluation of caries preventive programs. Which one to use depends on what question the evaluation strives to answer.

2.2 Perspective and time horizon of the evaluation

A health economic analysis can be performed from different perspectives. The healthcare and societal perspectives are the most used perspectives. The healthcare perspective covers all costs and effects that occur within the healthcare system such as clinic costs, material used, overhead costs, and so on. On the other hand, the societal perspective includes all costs and effects on society, regardless of who they impact. This perspective also considers indirect costs such as productivity loss and the need for informal care. Other perspectives may include the third-party payer, the clinic's, or the patient's perspective. Although there is no international agreement on what perspective to use [5], the health care and societal perspectives are the two most common in various national guidelines. Generally, the perspective used depends on the analysis's aim to provide information.

Most methodological guidelines in health economic evaluations agree that the analysis of costs and effects should have a time horizon that is long enough to reflect all significant differences in costs or outcomes related to the assessed program. This means that evaluations in, for example, prosthetics should include all future costs and effects related to the treatment, which may be a lifetime. The same applies to caries preventive programs, as this may affect the future incidence of new caries. However, the time horizon of the analysis should also be based on the level of data that exists and the uncertainty around that data. For instance, a decision-maker who considers a caries preventive program at school may not find a lifetime horizon to be relevant or trustworthy. Instead, a time horizon of, for example, 5 years could be more relevant.

It is essential to discount costs and effects that occur in the future annually to reflect their values at the time of the analysis. Although the discount rates may vary between guidelines, a rate of 3% per year is commonly used.

2.3 Costs

A program's cost goes beyond its price tag. The costs incurred are determined by the resources utilized and should be evaluated based on what those resources could have been used for elsewhere (the opportunity cost). It is best if all resources used are quantified and presented in natural units before being valued, to ensure transparency and transferability to other settings.

There are various ways to classify costs, but they are usually categorized as direct and indirect costs, or initial treatment and maintenance costs. Direct costs refer to resources such as dental personnel, all supplies and material used, dental clinic, administrative, and patient costs. Indirect costs are productivity losses linked to a treatment or health condition. Maintenance costs include all treatment costs that are not part of the initial treatment.

To accurately reflect the direct costs, the number of minutes the dental team spends on patients should be measured and valued. If a societal perspective is sought, all the time used by patients (and significant others, if applicable) should also be included. If the program requires multiple visits to the dental clinic, all time spent needs to be added up. The value of patients' time may be difficult to estimate, but it should reflect their opportunity cost. If the time used by patients would have otherwise been spent on paid production, the cost of having a person employed should be used (using the human capital method). If time off is used, the opportunity cost of this time off should be used, sometimes valued at 30% of paid production.

2.4 Outcomes

There are three different types of outcome measures that can be used to evaluate programs: clinical outcomes (including intermediate outcomes), measures of quality of life (QoL), and monetary outcomes. The choice of which measure to use depends on the purpose of the analysis.

Health economic evaluations allow for any kind of outcome measure to be used, but it is important that the chosen measure is relevant to the program being evaluated. For example, when evaluating a caries preventive program, the outcome measure should reflect the aims of the program. This might include factors such as the amount of caries, dmft/DMFT, pain, esthetics, or QoL.

The most commonly used outcome measure in healthcare programs is quality adjusted life year (QALY). This measure combines the value of a health state with the time spent in that state, providing scores on a scale with common anchor points. However, if QALY is to be used in caries preventive programs, it is important to consider whether it can capture oral health-related quality of life (OHRQoL) aspects [6].

It is necessary to choose outcome measures carefully, as they are used to inform decision-makers about the cost-effectiveness of proposed programs. If the chosen measure is not relevant to the decision-maker, then the analysis will not be useful. Therefore, it is important to consider the purpose of the analysis and who the decision-maker is when choosing an outcome measure.

3. Cost-effectiveness

If the evaluation's focus is on determining the cost-effectiveness of a program, then a cost-effectiveness analysis or cost-utility analysis is generally required. In this type of analysis, an incremental cost-effectiveness ratio (ICER) is calculated by dividing the difference in costs between at least two alternative programs with the difference in effects between the programs.

For instance, if program A costs \$100 per participant and causes 1 DMFT and program B costs \$50 per participant and causes 1.5 DMFT, this means that program A costs an additional \$50 and prevents 0.5 DMFT compared to program B. The ICER would then show that it costs an additional \$100 per DMFT prevented. Whether this is cost-effective or not depends on the willingness to pay to prevent DMFT. However, no such willingness-to-pay value exists, which makes it difficult to state if program A is cost-effective.

In the case where the outcome measure instead is QALY, the same program A may yield 0.80 QALY and program B 0.79 QALY, resulting in an increase of 0.01 QALY. The ICER of program A compared with program B would then be \$5000 per QALY gained (as shown in Eq. (1) below). Since QALY has been used in many studies and previous decisions, we know that the willingness to pay per QALY gained use to be much higher than \$5000. Therefore, program A can be considered cost-effective compared with program B.

Eq. (1). Calculation of the incremental cost-effectiveness ratio (ICER) of program a compared with program B is as shown below:

$$ICER = \frac{CostsA - CostsB}{EffectsA - EffectsB} = \frac{\$100 - \$50}{0.80\,QALY - 0.79\,QALY} = \frac{\$5000}{QALY} \qquad (1)$$

A cost-effectiveness analysis can be represented on a cost-effectiveness plane, as shown in **Figure 1** below. The ICER can be located in any of the four quadrants, A, B, C, or D. Only in quadrant A or D, it is straightforward to determine whether the program being evaluated is cost-effective, as it leads to either increased costs and lower effects or decreased costs and higher effects. However, in quadrant B or C, it depends

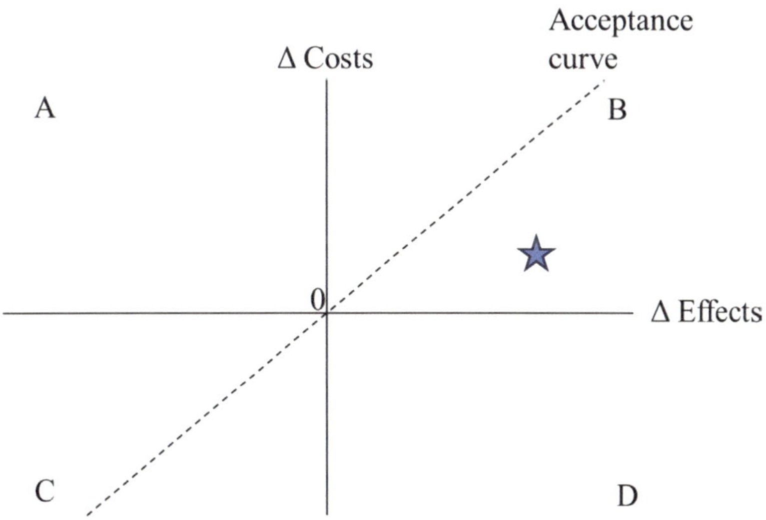

Figure 1.
The cost effectiveness plane. ★ = ICER of program a compared with program B.

on how much one is willing to pay for improved effects. The maximum willingness to pay for an additional effect can be shown on an acceptance curve, and all estimates below this curve are considered cost-effective. The star in the figure represents the potential ICER of program A compared with program B in Eq. (1) above, indicating that program A is deemed cost-effective.

4. Simulation and uncertainty

The main purpose of health economic analyses is to assist decision-makers in prioritizing between different programs or treatments. It is crucial to provide relevant and reliable information for this purpose, which often requires the use of simulation models and uncertainty analyses. In this part, we will briefly introduce these concepts.

4.1 Simulation models

Simulation involves creating models that replicate real-world scenarios to assess the potential impact of different programs on costs and outcomes. These models can be used to estimate the long-term costs and effects of a program and to synthesize available data from different sources [7]. Simulation models can also be used to generalize results from one context to another and to go from intermediate outcomes to other outcomes. There are three main types of simulation models used in health economic evaluations: decision trees, Markov models, and discrete event simulation.

Decision trees are the simplest type of model and are useful when the timeframe is short and when the process is not complex. For instance, a decision tree may be relevant in a caries preventive program to model how many people received caries with different programs. However, it is not suitable if you want to follow the caried tooth for a long time.

A Markov model is built around different states, in which a patient can stay or transfer to another state with certain probabilities. Such a model can be useful for dental caries as it may have a state of a sound tooth, another state with enamel caries, another one with dental caries, and so on. The model can run for many cycles, and the tooth (or the patient) may move between these states, causing costs or effects continuously, which can be summed up.

Finally, discrete event simulation is generally more advanced and requires data on a patient level. It allows the study of systems or processes whose state changes discretely over time.

4.2 Uncertainty

Uncertainty is a common challenge in health economic evaluations due to factors such as variations in patient outcomes, differences in care settings, and uncertainty in cost estimates. To ensure the reliability and application of evaluation results, it is important to address and quantify uncertainty. Sensitivity analysis is a fundamental tool for assessing the impact of uncertain parameters on the results of economic evaluations.

Sensitivity analysis involves varying key inputs and assumptions, such as treatment costs, disease prevalence, and treatment effectiveness, to identify the variables that have the greatest impact on outcomes. This process allows researchers to understand the strength of the results and make better-informed decisions.

There are different types of uncertainty that need to be dealt with differently. Parameter uncertainty relates to the fact that the true value is unknown, and this can be tested with statistical tests. Methodological uncertainty relates to all the methodological choices that must be made in an economic evaluation, and the significance of this can be tested by varying those choices. Structural uncertainty relates to how the decision is labeled, the comparator chosen, and the simulation model created. This type of uncertainty is often the most difficult to test.

Another type of sensitivity analysis is called bootstrapping, which is a statistical resampling technique used to estimate the uncertainty around cost and outcomes. It involves drawing multiple random samples with replacement from the original data to generate a distribution of cost and effectiveness estimates. This method provides confidence intervals around the point estimates, which help to understand the level of certainty in evaluation results.

Probabilistic sensitivity analysis goes further than traditional sensitivity analysis by including probability distributions for uncertain parameters. Instead of using single point estimates, a probabilistic sensitivity analysis assigns probability distributions to these parameters and performs thousands of simulation runs to generate a range of possible outcomes with associated probabilities.

In summary, simulation techniques and uncertainty analysis are important components of health economic evaluations. By using sophisticated simulation techniques and carefully addressing uncertainty, researchers can increase the credibility and utility of their findings. This can guide decision-makers in making evidence-based decisions that improve oral health outcomes and optimize resource allocation in dental care systems.

5. An example: fluoride varnishing program in school

Here follows an example of an economic evaluation of a caries preventive program and some aspects to consider. In this example, we evaluate a fictitious caries preventive program from a health economic perspective. A decision-maker is considering starting a fluoride varnishing program in schools for 12-year-old children. The main reason for this is that dental health is uneven, and high-risk children are difficult to reach. A program within schools has a high chance of capturing these hard-to-reach children. The comparator is no such program (treatment as usual).

We have chosen a cost-effectiveness analysis with the number of DMFT as the outcome measure. We have chosen a societal perspective and a time horizon of 5 years to capture the wide effects over a long time. The direct cost of each application has been found to be relatively low as a whole class can be treated within a short time. The cost includes the varnish used, the time used by dental personnel, and the costs for the person to get to the school. The cost of the involved children's time is set to zero as only a few minutes of school time are used.

Assuming the program would cost $50 per involved child and the varnish would lead to fewer DMFT compared to treatment as usual for children with moderate or high risk of caries, we need to study the relation between increased costs and improved outcomes to examine the cost-effectiveness. For children with low risk, the program only reduces DMFT by 0.1 compared to treatment as usual. For children with moderate or high risk, the number of DMFT is reduced by 0.4 and 1.0, respectively; see **Table 1**. This reduction in DMFT furthermore leads to reduced costs; that is why the cost difference in **Table 1** is lower than the cost of the program. However, the

Risk of caries	Long term results (5 years)		
	Low risk	Moderate risk	High risk
Cost difference ($)	45	30	10
DMFT difference	−0.1	−0.4	−1.0
ICER (cost per DMFT prevented)	450	75	10

Table 1.
Presentation of the incremental cost-effectiveness ratio of the example.

difference in cost is above zero for all risk groups, which means that the program will not lead to savings.

From **Table 1** we can see that the most favorable ICER is achieved for the group with a high risk of caries, but we could not state whether this is cost-effective or not as we do not know the willingness to pay per DMFT prevented.

If all the ICER of the risk groups from the example are plotted in the cost effectiveness plane, we might more easily see the difference between the groups; see **Figure 2**. If the maximum willingness-to-pay per DMFT prevented would be \$30, the program would only be cost-effective if directed toward the high caries risk group. If the maximum willingness-to-pay per DMFT prevented instead would be \$100, the program would be considered cost-effective also if directed toward those with a moderate risk. The program is probably not cost-effective if directed toward those with a low risk of caries. However, a school-based program would probably include all these groups, perhaps showing an average in risks close to the moderate risk group.

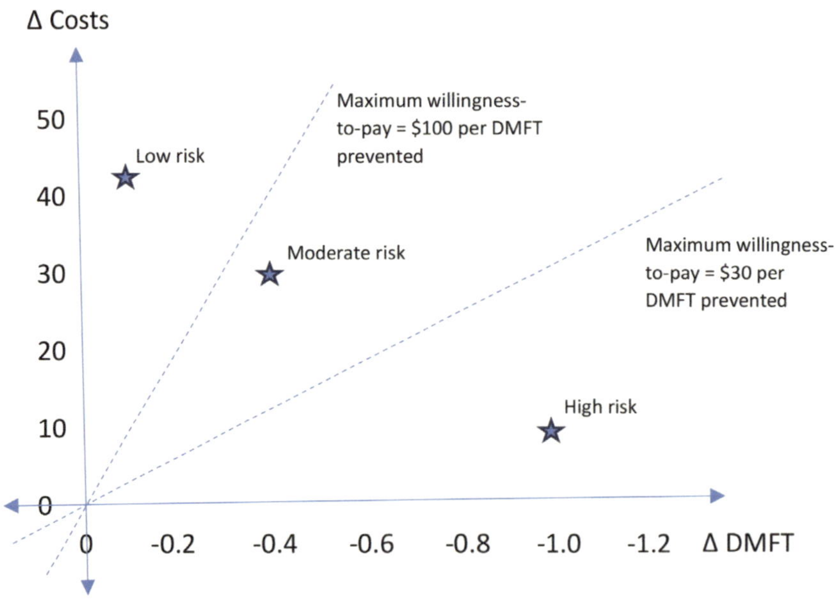

Figure 2.
Illustration of the cost-effectiveness of the example in a cost-effectiveness plane. ★ = ICER of program a compared with treatment as usual for three different risk groups.

6. Evidence of cost-effectiveness of caries preventive programs

There's plenty of evidence to suggest that caries preventive programs are cost-effective, as shown by various studies and health economic evaluations over the years; for example [8, 9]. However, there are some methodological weaknesses in many of the studies, and more research is needed to determine the value of such programs [10].

Most of the studies have focused on children with a high risk of caries, with fluoride varnish being the most common intervention. While these interventions have been successful and cost-effective, they are not directly applicable to the general population where caries incidence may be lower [8].

There are a few interventions that have been found to be effective and cost-efficient for the general population, such as risk-based interventions [11], frequency of dental check-ups [12], and taxes on sugar [13]. However, there is a lack of studies using QALY as the outcome measured, which makes it challenging for decision-makers to prioritize caries preventive interventions.

Water fluoridation is probably the most efficient program, which has been found to save costs and reduce caries [14]. However, many countries or regions have made this program illegal for different reasons.

Additionally, it is important to note that the cost-effectiveness of caries preventive programs can vary depending on several factors, including the target population, the specific intervention, the dental care setting, and regional healthcare costs. Therefore, conducting local or regional health economic evaluations is necessary to tailor preventive programs to the specific context and population. Overall, more research is needed to determine the cost-effectiveness of caries preventive programs and to improve their quality.

7. Discussion and conclusions

The efficient use of scarce resources is crucial in dentistry, which is why health economic evaluations are necessary. In this chapter, we have discussed various methods to achieve this objective. Health economic evaluations can also help prevent socioeconomic inequalities in dental health and support research in preventive dental care. We have also discussed the different types of health economic evaluations and identified cost-effectiveness analysis, including cost-utility analysis, as the most used ones. However, before selecting a particular methodology, it is crucial to define the decision problem clearly. This involves identifying the patients, intervention, comparator, and outcomes (PICO), as well as determining the perspective of the analysis and the cost-effectiveness threshold.

To ensure that the analysis covers all the critical aspects, it is recommended to use checklists [3]. Nevertheless, these checklists should be used in the context of their influence on the decision-making process, rather than the number of boxes ticked. Some items in the checklist may not be relevant to the decision problem, while other important aspects may be overlooked. For instance, the analysis's relevance to the decision problem, the inclusion of the best comparator, and the selection of the most relevant outcome measure are critical considerations.

It is essential to assess values that are important to patients when conducting health economic evaluations. The social function of esthetics, such as "kissing," may be more important to patients than the appearance of their teeth. Similarly, patients may view the chewing function as "meal joy" rather than merely a dental function [15].

To provide relevant health economic evaluations in dentistry, well-developed simulation models are also necessary. These models should analyze programs over an appropriate time horizon, combine sources from different areas, and explore total uncertainty. Additionally, health economic evaluations in dentistry would benefit from estimating QALY values for various dental health states.

In conclusion, assessing the cost-effectiveness of caries preventive programs is crucial in evidence-based decision-making in oral health. These evaluations provide valuable insights into the financial feasibility, value for money, and the long-term impact of preventive interventions. By understanding the cost-effectiveness of different programs, policymakers and dental professionals can develop sustainable, efficient, and equitable strategies to combat dental caries effectively and promote better oral health outcomes for populations.

Conflict of interest

The author declares no conflict of interest.

Author details

Thomas Davidson
Linköping University, Linköping, Sweden

*Address all correspondence to: thomas.davidson@liu.se

References

[1] Jain N, Dutt U, Radenkov I, Jain S. WHO's global oral health status report 2022: Actions, discussion and implementation. Oral Diseases. 2023:1-7. DOI: 10.1111/odi.14516

[2] Listl S, Galloway J, Mossey PA, Marcenes W. Global economic impact of dental diseases. Journal of Dental Research. 2015;**94**(10):1355-1361

[3] Drummond M, Sculpher M, Claxton K, Stoddart G, Torrance G. Methods for the Economic Evaluation of Health Care Programmes. 4th ed. Oxford: Oxford University Press; 2015

[4] Sullivan SD, Mauskopf JA, Augustovski F, Jaime Caro J, Lee KM, Minchin M, et al. Budget impact analysis-principles of good practice: Report of the ISPOR 2012 budget impact analysis good practice II task force. Value in Health. 2014;**17**(1):5-14

[5] EUnetHTA Joint Action 2 Work Package 7 Subgroup 3, Heintz E, Gerber-Grote A, Ghabri S, Hamers F, Prevolnik Rupel V, et al. It there a European view on health economic evaluations? Results from a synopsis of methodlogical guidelines used in the EUnetHTA partner countries. PharmacoEconomics. 2015;**34**(1):59-76

[6] Davidson T. Measuring effectiveness for use in economic evaluations in oral health. In: Zaror C, Marino R, editors. Introduction to Economic Evaluation in Oral Health Care. Cham, Switzerland: Springer; 2022

[7] De La Puente C, Marino R, Espinoza-Espinoza G. Aspects of decision modelling for economic evaluation in oral health care. In: Zaror C, Marino R, editors. Introduction to Economic Evaluation in Oral Health Care. Cham, Switzerland: Springer; 2022

[8] Davidson T, Blomma C, Bagesund M, Krevers B, Vall M, Warnberg Gerdin E, et al. Cost-effectiveness of caries preventive interventions - a systematic review. Acta Odontologica Scandinavica. 2020;**79**(4):1-12

[9] Eow J, Duane B, Solaiman A, Hussain U, Lemasney N, Ang R, et al. What evidence do economic evaluations in dental care provide? A scoping review. Community Dental Health. 2019;**36**(2):118-125

[10] Rogers HJ, Rodd HD, Vermaire JH, Stevens K, Knapp R, El Yousfi S, et al. A systematic review of the quality and scope of economic evaluations in child oral health research. BMC Oral Health. 2019;**19**(1):132

[11] Warren E, Curtis B, Jia N, Evans W. The caries management system: Updating cost-effectiveness with 4-year posttrial data. International Journal of Technology Assessment in Health Care. 2016;**32**(3):107-115

[12] Davenport C, Elley K, Salas C, Taylor-Weetman CL, Fry-Smith A, Bryan S, et al. The clinical effectiveness and cost-effectiveness of routine dental checks: A systematic review and economic evaluation. Health Technology Assessment. 2003;**7**(7):1-127: p. iii-v

[13] Jevdjevic M, Trescher AL, Rovers M, Listl S. The caries-related cost and effects of a tax on sugar-sweetened beverages. Public Health. 2019;**169**:125-132

[14] Marino R, Zaror C. Economic evaluations in water-fluoridation: A scoping review. BMC Oral Health. 2020;**20**(1):115

[15] Nordenram G, Davidson T, Gynther G, Helgesson G, Hultin M, Jemt T, et al. Qualitative studies of patients' perceptions of loss of teeth, the edentulous state and prosthetic rehabilitation: A systematic review with meta-synthesis. Acta Odontologica Scandinavica. 2013;**71**(3-4):937-951